AF709722

Multicultural Counseling in a Divided and Traumatized Society

Recent Titles in
Contributions in Psychology

Counseling in the Asia-Pacific Region
Abdul Halim Othman and Amir Awang, editors

What Wrongdoers Deserve: The Moral Reasoning Behind Responses to Misconduct
R. Murray Thomas and Ann Diver-Stamnes

Using Bibliotherapy in Clinical Practice: A Guide to Self-Help Books
John T. Pardeck

Modern Perspectives on John B. Watson and Classical Behaviorism
James T. Todd and Edward K. Morris, editors

Worlds of Common Sense: Equality, Identity, and Two Modes of Impulse Management
Pauline Nichols Pepinsky

The Five Stages of Culture Shock: Critical Incidents Around the World
Paul Pedersen

Modern Perspectives on B. F. Skinner and Contemporary Behaviorism
James T. Todd and Edward K. Morris, editors

Chaos Theory in Psychology
Frederick David Abraham and Albert R. Gilgen, editors

Classifying Reactions to Wrongdoing
R. Murray Thomas

Prevent, Repent, Reform, Revenge: A Study in Adolescent Moral Development
Ann C. Diver-Stamnes and R. Murray Thomas

Post-Soviet Perspectives on Russian Psychology
Vera Koltsova, Yuri Oleinik, Albert R. Gilgen, and Carol K. Gilgen, editors

Multicultural Counseling in a Divided and Traumatized Society

The Meaning of Childhood and Adolescence in South Africa

Joyce Hickson
and Susan Kriegler

Foreword by Paul Pedersen

Contributions in Psychology, Number 32
Paul Pedersen, Series Advisor

GREENWOOD PRESS
Westport, Connecticut • London

Library of Congress Cataloging-in-Publication Data

Hickson, Joyce.
Multicultural counseling in a divided and traumatized society : the meaning of childhood and adolescence in South Africa / Joyce Hickson, Susan Kriegler ; foreword by Paul Pedersen
p. cm.—(Contributions in psychology, ISSN 0736–2714 ; no. 32)
Includes bibliographical references and index.
ISBN 0–313–28554–3 (alk. paper)
1. Child mental health services—South Africa. 2. Cross-cultural counseling—South Africa. 3. Counselor and client—South Africa. 4. Apartheid—South Africa—Psychological aspects. 5. Child mental health—South Africa. 6. Children—South Africa—Social conditions. I. Kriegler, Susan. II. Title. III. Series.
RJ502.S6H53 1996
362.2'0968—dc20 95–41697

British Library Cataloguing in Publication Data is available.

Copyright © 1996 by Joyce Hickson and Susan Kriegler

All rights reserved. No portion of this book may be reproduced, by any process or technique, without the express written consent of the publisher.

Library of Congress Catalog Card Number: 95–41697
ISBN: 0–313–28554–3
ISSN: 0736–2714

First published in 1996

Greenwood Press, 88 Post Road West, Westport, CT 06881
An imprint of Greenwood Publishing Group, Inc.

Printed in the United States of America

The paper used in this book complies with the Permanent Paper Standard issued by the National Information Standards Organization (Z39.48–1984).

10 9 8 7 6 5 4 3 2 1

To our students

Contents

Series Foreword

South Africa has much to teach us in other countries about our own apartheid and our very limited success in dealing with it. As each country and culture becomes aware of the power of multicultural awareness as a bottom-up, consumer-driven revolution of modern society, it becomes important for them to learn from the others about what works and what does not work. South Africa has provided a laboratory of both the problems and the opportunities in multicultural awareness. This book seeks to guide the counselor through each learning experience toward increased multicultural awareness, not only about South Africa but, by extrapolation, about other countries and cultures as well.

Culture provides the foundation of identity, and therefore, the basis of all communication. Each behavior is displayed in a cultural context of learned values, expectations and perceptions of reality. Multicultural awareness, therefore, is the process of learning about the culturally learned assumptions that control behavior and the perception of reality. Each person's decisions are based on those culturally learned perceptions. Multicultural awareness is not merely learning about exotic societies in far away places, but also about the sources of assumptions and the contrasting assumptions of culturally different others.

South Africa provides an ideal example by which to examine the effect of those learned assumptions on multicultural awareness, because the different culturally learned assumptions were especially well-defined throughout society by explicit and precise rules. South Africa also provides a multicultural laboratory by which to examine the effect of explicit cultural differences so that we can learn more about implicit cultural differences in our own cultures.

Hickson and Kriegler do a masterful job of testing what we know—or think we know—about multicultural awareness against the reality of modern South Africa, both before and after apartheid. President Mandella and Bishop Desmond Tutu, for example, understand the importance of culture in the South African setting because they have had to manage both the problems and the opportunities of multiculturalism. We counselors and counselor educators are aware of the problems created by multiculturalism and often treat culture as a barrier to understanding. The leaders of modern South Africa, including President Mandella and Bishop Desmond Tutu, recognize the social and political opportunities of multiculturalism. There are counseling opportunities as well, which are addressed in this book.

Culture is the only construct in the social sciences that makes it possible for two people to disagree—in their behaviors, for example—without one necessarily being right and the other wrong when they are from different cultures. Multicultural awareness makes it possible to value both the ways we are similar *and* the ways we are different. The similarities of common-ground expectations for trust, respect, fairness and success require the cooperation of people who have attached different, and sometimes conflicting, behaviors to those shared expectations. The multicultural model, therefore, is the ideal basis for national, social and political development in South Africa. From the applications of this multicultural model in South Africa, we can better learn how it applies elsewhere.

This volume describes how that common ground can become the basis for successful multicultural counseling, not only in South Africa, but elsewhere as well. In the years of isolation, psychology developed independently in South Africa, generating new and uniquely original solutions to familiar problems. The psychological importance of context clearly emerges to demonstrate the psychological opportunities of indigenous multiculturalism.

Each of the well-defined and carefully bounded cultural groups of South Africa are examined in terms of their own indigenous context, as it is similar, and also different, from other cultural contexts. Because culture was recognized as central and fundamental to South African society—rather than marginal and peripheral as in European and American societies—the managing of multicultural awareness is explicit and direct, even in its injustices. The relationship of "settler" societies with one another and with the indigenous people is defined primarily in cultural terms, and counseling services have had to define themselves around the centrality of a cultural reality.

As multiculturalism becomes more central, fundamental and explicit in European and American societies, and less marginalized, we also will need to learn the implications of multicultural awareness. Hickson and Kriegler provide valuable guidelines for the counseling profession in the context of South African society, where multicultural awareness has been a central sociopolitical phenomenon for some time. The book is an optimistic treatment of multicultural awareness as a force toward a stronger and healthier society in which cooperation replaces contention and the shared common-ground expectations provide a safe context for disagreements. We need to learn more of what South Africans already know regarding multicultural awareness. Hickson and Kriegler go to great effort to help us learn in this book.

—Paul Pedersen
Syracuse University

Preface

The purpose of this book is to provide students, teachers and professionals with a conceptual and applied resource for working with culturally diverse groups. Using South Africa as a case example, the book focuses on the worldwide challenge to the helping professions to contribute toward creating harmony in multiethnic societies. In addressing the issues of conflict with respect to prejudice, racism, violence and civil war, any society may be placed on a continuum. The position of a society on this continuum is not fixed, as the dynamics and processes of conflict are not static. For example, certain multicultural societies experience group conflict at subliminal and covert levels whereas other societies express polarization by way of overt violence. Therefore, any multicultural society may be located on a continuum, and the directionality of its movement toward either conflict resolution or eruption may be predicted. South Africa today, with the drafting of a new constitution that will enfranchise all its citizens, is negotiating and moving toward a greater degree of multiethnic harmony. Nonetheless, because the scars of apartheid will remain for a long time, the present text describes childhood and adolescence in a society that has been severely divided and traumatized by institutionalized racism.

This book describes current counseling and educational issues in South Africa and a myriad of disorders that are the effects of structural inequality. A systemic view that places the individual in a social context has been adopted. Childhood and adolescence have been located within the wider social, economic and political arena and within the framework of two societies: the privileged and nonprivileged sectors.

The book is divided into five sections. Part I, "Foundations," provides an overview and rationale for a cross-cultural counseling approach and describes the distinct focus of the text. Part II, "World-View and Identity," describes ethnocultural considerations and the world-view of Africans, Afrikaners, Indians and coloreds as group members within the South African society. Part III, "Psychological Trauma in Childhood and Adolescence," portrays the large number of children whose physical and psychological needs are unmet and the current youth revolt against an unjust social and educational system. Part IV, "Educational and Mental Health Issues," describes a new paradigm for use in multicultural school settings. Finally, the Afterword, "Hope and Reconciliation in the 'New' South Africa," presents a new role for mental health workers and suggests the use of creative, imaginative and resourceful strategies responsive to the unique needs of a divided and culturally diverse society.

The authors express appreciation to Paul Pedersen, Series Advisor, and hope this volume will provide a substantive starting place for helping professionals to increase their knowledge and skills in providing help to the peoples from different ethnocultural traditions in South Africa.

Part I

Foundations

Chapters 1 and 2 describe cultural encapsulation and the impact of cross-cultural variables on the relationship, process and outcome of counseling and psychotherapy. These chapters focus on the need to prepare culturally effective counselors and the importance of the therapist's sensitivity to culture in terms of the three interrelated areas of knowledge, awareness and skill. Cross-cultural counseling is located within the broader South African sociopolitical environment and the chapters also discuss how a history of oppression, discrimination and racism have affected the way non-white constituencies perceive the mental health profession. Although specific barriers to multicultural counseling are acknowledged, a multicultural perspective is presented and provides a conceptual framework that recognizes the diversity of a plural society while suggesting bridges of shared concern. The multicultural approach explains behavior in terms of culturally learned perspectives as well as common-ground universals. The fact remains, however, that no individual can be totally "culture free." The helping professional must be aware of certain cultural constructs that may have shaped the client as well as individual differences that are personal and unique. A clear need exists for comprehensive multicultural training for counselors, guidance personnel, psychologists, social workers, teachers and other helping professionals as South Africa moves away from racism and oppression toward the new South Africa that celebrates diversity.

1

Issues and Concepts of Cross-Cultural Counseling: Implications for the South African Context

> The price one pays for living in a color-bar society is a cauterization of the human heart, a coarseness of feelings, a fear that destroys all relationships (Gordimer, 1954, p. 95).

South Africa is a land of contrasts. Geographically there is Mediterranean coastland, snow-covered mountains, parkland, forests, desert—almost every kind of vegetational zone except arctic tundra or tropical rainforest. The peoples of South Africa are equally varied. South Africa is a complex tapestry of differing races and ethnic groups—the world in microcosm.

The four major population groups in South Africa are white, African, Asian (Indian) and colored (people of mixed descent). Within each of these major groups members often differ considerably from one another. Despite these contrasts, however, the four groups also have common cultural characteristics.

CULTURE

Brislin (1990) alludes to the importance of cultural identity as follows:

> Culture refers to the widely shared ideals, values, formation and use of categories, assumptions about life and goal directed activities that become unconsciously or subconsciously accepted as "right" and "correct" by people who identify themselves as members of a society. . . . A society is sometimes a country (e.g., Japan), sometimes a more delimited segment of society (e.g., the middle class in the United States) and sometimes an ethnic group within a large country (e.g., Polish Americans or Palestinian Arabs living in Israel. (P. 11)

The perception of rules and group norms, roles and values are all aspects of culture. Cultural assumptions and traditions are indelibly imprinted on each individual. Herr (1987) acknowledges their legacy as follows:

> the continuing intergenerational effects that family background transmits or reinforces through formation of values; orientation to the past, present and future, ways of viewing and interacting with strangers and persons beyond the family boundaries; interpretations of obligations and responsibilities to others; views of work, marriage and childbearing; problem definition and appropriate solutions, or ways of coping with a cultural identity. Such traditions persist for long periods in people's concepts of who they are and the behavioral norms to which they subscribe. (Pp. 99–100)

Accordingly, each individual is embedded within a particular context and inherits cultural patterns of thought and action. This frame of reference becomes a world-view and includes attitudes, folkways, behavior styles, values and traditions. A person's orientation serves as a lens through which experience is filtered and a reference point from which individuals encounter the world, themselves and life. Culture becomes the glue that binds people together in the preservation of a society. Cultural identity cannot be separated from the development of the individual's personality and becomes an integral part of the way he or she constructs reality. As Segall, Dason, Berry and Poortinga (1990) suggest: "There may well come a time when we will no longer speak of cross-cultural psychology as such. The basic premise of this field—that to understand human behavior we must study it in its socio-cultural context—may become so widely accepted that all psychology will be inherently cultural" (p. 352).

Accordingly, culture reflects the subjective orientation toward life that individuals have. It serves as the lens through which individuals make decisions and manifest various behaviors. Culture is a binding element that defines and unifies various populations. Cultural awareness enables the individual to understand variations between different groups of people while understanding his or her own "culture baggage" and subjective perspective as well.

MULTICULTURAL PERSPECTIVES

Pedersen (1991) has recognized the importance of cultural awareness and has described the multicultural revolution in counseling as follows:

> We are moving toward a generic theory of multiculturalism as a "fourth force" position, complementing the other three forces of psychodynamic, behavioral and humanistic explanations of human behavior. The label of fourth force emphasizes that multiculturalism is relevant throughout the field of counseling as a generic rather than an exotic perspective. (P. 6)

This multicultural perspective is particularly fitting in South Africa because it provides a conceptual framework that recognizes the diversity of a plural society while, at the same time, suggesting bridges of shared concern that bind culturally different persons to one another.

It is very important to realize that although there are culture-specific characteristics of various groups in South Africa, there are general cultural features that are shared by all people and which unite those living in the same country. Given South Africa's history, there is a danger in emphasizing separatism in ways that are divisive and disunifying. The focus on the cultural identity of the individual need not be at the expense of other influential agents such as individual differences and universal tenets of humanness. In order to understand the complex pluralism that exists in South African society, both within-group differences as well as between-group differences must be acknowledged. Multicultural relationships must be viewed as representing a myriad of factors.

In explaining this perspective Pedersen (1991) made the following observations:

> The multicultural perspective combines the extremes of relativism by explaining behavior both in terms of those culturally learned perspectives that are unique to a particular culture and in the search for common ground universals that are shared across cultures. The "melting pot" metaphor made the mistake of overemphasizing universal common ground generalizations that are shared across cultures to the neglect of culturally unique perspectives. The phenomena of racism, sexism, ageism and other exclusionary perspectives make the mistake of overemphasizing the culturally unique perspective while neglecting those common ground universals and within-group differences that are shared across cultures. (P. 6)

It cannot be assumed that all persons from the same ethnic group are alike, for not all Africans have the same experience nor do all Indians, or coloreds or Afrikaners. It is wrong to assume that any particular group is unimodal in its perspective. Individual differences exist among clients from every cultural group. However, such an individual has still been influenced by being a part of a group with certain ethnographic variables such as ethnicity, language, religion, history and common ancestry. No individual can be totally "culture free." The helping professional must be aware of certain cultural constructs that may have shaped the client as well as individual differences that are personal and unique. Helping professionals who ignore the influence of a client's cultural context are unlikely to interpret a client's behavior accurately. Cross-cultural awareness ensures the use of more accurate approaches to differences across groups in a pluralistic population. From this perspective a client's intended meaning in light of his/her cultural framework can be better understood. Accurately perceiving a problem from the client's vantage point is necessary in order to have a successful helping relationship.

CULTURAL PERSPECTIVES VERSUS INDIVIDUAL DIFFERENCES

According to Brislin (1990) cultural perspectives reflect the following dimensions:

1. The part of a way of life that people make
2. Ideas transmitted from generation to generation
3. Identifiable childhood experiences resulting in internalized values
4. Socialization of children into adults
5. Consistent patterns of concepts and practices
6. Cultural patterns that one maintains despite slipups in the system
7. Feelings of helplessness or bewilderment that result when cultural patterns are changed

The skilled professional must be able to differentiate between the individual differences the client brings and the cultural perspective that may be operating. It is also very important for counselors to understand client world-views that are based on culturally different assumptions so that individual behavior can be understood and interpreted. Rather than trying to displace traditional theories of counseling—psychodynamic, humanistic and cognitive-behavioral—multi-cultural approaches should complement them. Accordingly, any counseling theory can be adapted to fit unique cultural perspectives. Unless multiculturally adapted approaches are used, the helping professional will be operating from an exclusionary perspective and will be guilty of an ethnocentric viewpoint.

CULTURAL ENCAPSULATION

Wrenn (1962, 1985) identified the dangers of cultural encapsulation as follows:

1. The helping professional defines reality according to one set of cultural stereotypes.
2. The world-view of the helper is assumed to be the only superior and legitimate world-view. Any cultural variations expressed in clients are not legitimate.
3. Assumptions are held unquestioningly and without the scrutiny of rationality.
4. Helpers are technique oriented, use a self-reference criterion and do not evaluate other viewpoints.

Pedersen (1987) also describes the dangers of cultural encapsulation: "The majority of people in the world accept a non-Western perspective. Despite that numerical reality, many social scientists, including psychologists, depend on textbooks, research findings, and entirely on assumptions specific in European and American culture" (p. 16).

Pedersen (1987) also enumerates ten assumptions in counseling that reflect cultural bias on the part of the helper:

1. Assumptions regarding normal behavior and the assumption that the definition of normal is more or less universal across social, cultural and economic or political backgrounds. What is considered normal will change according to the situation, the cultural background of a person or persons being judged and the time during which a behavior is being displayed or observed.

2. Emphasis on individualism rather than the welfare of the family, group and society.
3. A narrow perspective of psychology and counseling rather than integrating the findings of disciplines such as anthropology, sociology, theology, medicine and the like.
4. Dependence on abstract words in their theoretical formulations and practices and a lack of cognizance that such abstractions lose their meaning or take on different meanings when used outside the cultural context in which they were generated.
5. Overemphasis on independence rather than an appreciation that in many cultures dependence is regarded as healthy and necessary.
6. Neglect of the client's support system and the elimination of family, peers, and indigenous healers in the helping process and treatment plan.
7. Dependence on linear thinking and cause and effect relationships rather than nonlinear and circular modes which are used by certain cultures.
8. Focusing on changing the individual instead of the system and being an agent of the prevailing social system.
9. Neglect of history and an emphasis on the here and now. Many cultures have a past orientation and a sense of history about their people. They see themselves as being intimately connected to their ancestors. This orientation is neglected.
10. Cultural encapsulation and a closed biased system that promotes domination by an elitist group.

In essence, in being culturally encapsulated the helper uses one lens to evaluate all human behavior. Adaptation and alternative ways of thinking are rejected. As Hoare (1991) notes:

> The particular lens of our culture, and of our position in it, imparts a bias from which there is no escape. . . . We must accept that we are not objective . . . and that there is a direct relationship between the depth of understanding of our (conscious and unconscious) biases and our ability to unimposingly hear and help those who do not share our culturally derived views. (P. 51)

Accordingly, it is no wonder that the culturally different client may approach the counseling situation wondering, "What makes you, a counselor-therapist, any different from all the others out there who have oppressed and discriminated against me?" (Sue & Sue, 1990, p. 6). Indeed Ponterretto and Casas (1991) have provided evidence that "the majority of traditionally trained counselors operate from a culturally biased and encapsulated framework which results in the provision of culturally conflicting and even oppressive counseling treatments" (pp. 7–8).

A clear need exists for comprehensive multicultural training for counselors, guidance personnel, psychologists, social workers, teachers and other helping professionals as South Africa moves away from racism and oppression toward the new South Africa that celebrates diversity and a nonracial democracy. There is a clear need to identify one's own cultural disposition as well as the need to give validity to other cultural perspectives. Becoming aware and understanding one's own cultural assumptions can facilitate an awareness of alternative values and ways of being. Learning to compare one's own cultural perspective with that of a person from another culture can enlarge one's own perspective and teach the individual a great deal about his or her own cultural biases. After shifting to a multicultural perspective, no culture can be viewed as superior when compared to the culture of another group. All cultures are coequal in the sense that there are many valid and different ways of being human.

CROSS-CULTURAL COUNSELING CONCERNS

Research studies on cross-cultural variables have focused on the effects of race or ethnicity on the relationship, process and outcome of counseling and psychotherapy. Many mental health professionals, consequently, concluded that racial or ethnic factors had important implications for the client-counselor interpersonal alliance. Vontress (1969) specified six possible racial barriers: (1) racial attitudes, (2) ignorance of the client's background, (3) language, (4) client's unfamiliarity with therapy, (5) client's low self-disclosure and (6) sex and race taboos. In another study, Vontress (1979) also suggested that racial differences in the therapeutic encounter served to interfere with establishing and maintaining rapport. Extending Vontress' work, Padilla, Ruiz and Alveraz (1975) identified three major factors as hindering the formation of a good therapeutic relationship: (1) language barriers, (2) class-bound values and (3) culture-bound values.

While it is generally recognized that a number of factors such as client-counselor match, therapist characteristics and appropriateness of interventions utilized may act as impediments to the counseling process, certain obstacles are also present when monocultural rather than cross-cultural practices are utilized in any culturally diverse society. Cross-cultural researchers (Sue & Sue, 1977) have identified the following difficulties:

1. Racial and ethnic factors are not only barriers to the delivery of helping services, but also may lead to alienation or an inability to develop trust or rapport with the culturally different.
2. Such factors may result in the underutilization of mental health services by Third World clients.
3. Racial and ethnic factors may also lead to premature client termination.

In the late 1960s and early 1970s many articles were written relating to racial and ethnic minority group counseling. Different theories, models and techniques were increasingly devised for overcoming barriers, counseling blacks, counseling across cultures and counseling in a multicultural school setting. It was generally asserted by researchers that therapists should adopt an eclectic approach and be more action oriented, directive and concrete in order to better meet the needs of the culturally different client. Such needs were assumed to include feelings of low self-esteem, hostility, fear, distress, self-hatred and self-pity. Midgette and Meggert (1991) identified specific barriers to multicultural counseling as follows:

1. Counselor-client incongruent expectations about counseling
2. Counselor overemphasis on verbal self-disclosure
3. Counselor overemphasis on abstract and non–problem-solving strategies
4. Counselor use of monolingual orientation
5. Value placed in counseling on long-range goals and the future
6. Lack of understanding of whole person
7. Lack of understanding of the social focus and environment of the client and how this effects problems of living
8. Inability to understand client's nonverbal messages and behavior

Although both problem definition and suggestions of intervention techniques were intended to be helpful, the current cross-cultural perspective has been criticized for depicting stereotypes and caricatures of individuals. Furthermore, a certain dissatisfaction was expressed among the ranks of helping professionals who disagreed with a cross-cultural focus and stressed, instead, the universality of suffering and confusion in the human psyche. Maslow (1971), for example, expressed the belief that therapists who are able to empathize with clients on the human rather than the cultural level will be able to identify and share experiences in spite of differences in cultural or racial background. Maslow's position represents a belief in the continuity of human experience regardless of ethnic differences and is echoed by Sullivan's (1953) postulate: "We are all much more simply human than otherwise" (p. 322).

Despite the concern that has been voiced about the dangers of "cultural stereotyping," there continues to be an increasing orientation to the needs of culturally different clients and to racial and ethnic variables within the therapeutic process. In a benchmark position statement, the American Psychological Association (APA) sponsored a conference in Vail, Colorado (Korman, 1974), which strongly recommended that the counseling of persons of culturally diverse backgrounds by persons who are not trained or competent to work with such groups should be regarded as unethical. This recommendation was intended to make knowledge of culture a direct, practical concern for the majority of practicing clinical psychologists, and, by implication, all mental health practitioners.

Cultural sensitivity is currently considered a prerequisite to professional competence. Ahia (1984) summarized this viewpoint: "Cross-cultural counseling researchers and practitioners need to approach their work from the premise that cultures are not comparatively "better" or "worse," "superior" or "inferior," "meaningful" or "meaningless," rather that each culture is different and excitingly pregnant" (p. 341).

Accordingly, instead of ignoring cultural variables, a common concern now is to be sensitive enough to recognize, appreciate and respect similarities and differences in clients of diverse cultures.

Pedersen (1978b) broadens the idea of cross-cultural variables to include not only ethnic factors but almost all differences. These include the following variables: "If we consider the value perspective of age, sex role, lifestyle, socio-economic status and other special affiliations as cultural, then we may well conclude that all counseling is to some extent cross-cultural" (p. 480).

CONCLUSION

All differences between human beings in South Africa are not necessarily cultural. Persons from the same ethnic background may experience the culture differently. It cannot be asserted that all black men in South Africa are alike, for example. No particular group is unimodal in its cultural perspective. As this chapter noted, cultural aspects can be distinguished from individual differences by seven indicators (Brislin, 1990). A distinction between individual differences and cultural differences is important and must be adopted in order to have an accurate multicultural perspective. For example, skin color may represent an individual difference, yet culturally may come to symbolize more than one's racial identity. "Color" may symbolize significant connotative social meanings for particular societies. Social definition may be given to physical features and may determine social codes of interaction and conduct, regulating distance among individuals in a color-caste society. Individual characteristics and cultural predispositions must not be confused. In understanding individual versus cultural differences, it must be remembered that all individuals are embedded in societies that forge their identities. Individuals within any given society both absorb and reflect the culture. In this sense one's identity is group-based to a certain extent. However, one's personal identity also includes individual and unique characteristics not to be confused with cultural determinants. In order to understand an individual, the helping professional must be cognizant of how the individual may have been shaped by his or her cultural origin, yet also understand that the personal identity of the individual has unique characteristics.

2

Psychology in South Africa

Multicultural counseling and training issues have been discussed by counselors and psychologists for a number of years. Due to an increased awareness of multicultural concerns on the part of therapeutic practitioners, numerous approaches for training effective multicultural counselors have been proposed. In the South African context the professional must seriously consider the influence of the social environment and the functioning of social institutions as influential agents on human behavior.

Pedersen (1985) summarized the process of increasing a therapist's sensitivity to culture in terms of three interrelated areas: (1) knowledge, (2) awareness and (3) skills. Gaining knowledge of an individual's culture thus enhances a therapist's awareness of using culturally appropriate skills. It is also important that the therapist knows when and how to structure the counseling according to the individual's cultural frame of reference. Without a framework of cultural reference and appropriate skills, the therapist is left to respond intuitively and spontaneously, but perhaps not always in a culturally effective manner.

Many of the cross-cultural training models which have been developed share the following characteristics:

1. A basic assumption that an individual's ethnic or cultural background significantly influences his or her world-view and the way in which he or she experiences and understands life and its problems
2. An emphasis on learning about various cultural groups (i.e., cultural world-views) so that there is some understanding of how an individual from a particular group may experience life and its problems

3. A focus on teaching counseling skills and interventions appropriate for use with members of various ethnic groups

Many of the models also encourage self-exploration and an awareness that practitioners are themselves a product of their own culture, class, language and experience. From this perspective there is a need to be aware and accepting of one's own cultural baggage and how it can impact on the helping encounter. Therapists need to examine and evaluate the relevance of their particular framework and how it can operate as a potential source of conflict in the helping encounter. Encapsulated theories and practices should be discarded and more appropriate interventions used that are grounded in respect for diverse clients' cultural beliefs and values. In sum, both a sensitivity to the possession of an ethnocentric world-view and an awareness of how this will block authentic interaction are needed. A system of self-examination that promotes the practitioner's awareness of self-racism and others' cultural identities is needed. The therapist, then, is essentially in the position of being a cultural broker—a facilitator ideally without prejudice—of the individual's search for self and development of his or her own true potential. The therapist with cultural expertise must also remove any blindfold to the social ills within a society and must become proactive in relation to the human condition of those seeking help. In sum, the cross-cultural therapist should be able to meet the world and the people in it in depth and to share in the same reality in a collaborative endeavor to effect change.

THE SOUTH AFRICAN CONTEXT

It is thus clear that publications highlighting the need for all therapists to be culturally skilled have proliferated. Five general characteristics describing culturally effective therapists have been proposed (Sue & Sue, 1990):

1. Therapists should have an understanding of their own values and assumptions about human behavior and be able to recognize and accept values different from their own as legitimate.
2. Therapists must have an awareness of the generic characteristics of counseling and their relation to class and culture.
3. Therapists need to act on the basis of a critical analysis and understanding of their own conditioning, that of their clients, and the sociopolitical system of which they are a part.
4. Therapists need to become culturally aware, to understand the basis for their world-views and to understand and accept the possible legitimacy of world-views different from their own.
5. Culturally effective therapists are truly eclectic in their counseling and are able to generate the widest repertoire of microcounseling skills appropriate to the lifestyle of their individual client.

The issue of whether current psychological service is relevant to the South African social context has been steadily debated in recent years, with several mental health professionals concluding that psychology is irrelevant to the nature and needs of the majority of black people (Anonymous, 1986; Dawes, 1986; Holdstock, 1981; Jordaan & Jordaan, 1984; Strumpfer, 1981; Turton, 1986; Van Schoor, 1986). This debate has been pursued from diverse ideological standpoints focusing on (1) the examination of psychology as a scientific discipline (Ivey, 1986; Moll, 1983), (2) the translation of this discipline into counseling practice (Anonymous, 1986; Dawes, 1986; Holdstock, 1979; Strumpfer, 1981; Turton, 1986), (3) the ensuing role of psychologists in South Africa (Cloete, Pillay & Swart, 1986; Lazarus, 1986; Van Schoor, 1986) and (4) the need to reassess training (Dawes, 1986; Holdstock, 1981; Lazarus, 1986; Psychology in Society Editorial, 1986; Steyn, 1985; Swartz, Dowdall & Swartz, 1986).

Traditional fields of application, such as clinical psychology, have come under attack for being inappropriate for black clients. Consequently, alternative psychological services for working with African people have been propounded and it has been suggested that psychologists take up such roles as outreach liaison, consultant, ombudsman and facilitator of indigenous support systems. The need to include informal help and indigenous healing has received considerable attention and support from South African researchers (Buhrmann, 1977; Holdstock, 1979; Kruger, 1974).

Widespread support has also been given to the need to place South African psychology in its political, social and economic context (Cloete, Pillay, and Swart 1986; Dawes, 1986; Lazarus, 1986; Psychology in Society Editorial, 1983, 1986). In this regard, community psychology has attained considerable relevance for research in the present South African situation in that it relates human behavior to the total environmental context in which it occurs: social, economic, demographic, urban/rural, cultural and political (Lazarus, 1986). Another promising area of research is the cross-fertilization of theories of culture and environment that examine environmental functioning, cultural evolution and adaptation to the environment (Retief, 1986). Finally, Biesheuvel (1987) states that the interracial situation in South Africa is extremely complex and recommends that several variables be considered as areas of conflict, including prejudice, fear and economic exploitation on the part of the dominant white culture, as well as religious, national, economic, class, cultural and familial factors on the part of the client group.

The need to devise and provide alternative relevant help in South Africa is rooted in the knowledge that the common constructs of psychology are Western in origin and tend to be culture bound and culture blind, and thus not necessarily meaningful in other cultures (Biesheuvel, 1987). Abdi (1975) believes that the concepts of psychology, including its theories and methods, as understood by Westerners, are alien to the thinking of Africans. For instance, Western approaches fail to consider the spiritual dimension in the lives of the majority of the black population, and Western techniques, with a few exceptions, are culturally too different to offer a meaningful psychological approach toward healing. In addition, and consistent with Biesheuvel's (1987) idea that it is impossible to eliminate values from an analysis of human behavior, is the realization that a Western psychological analysis is uncharacteristic of the behavior of blacks, and that the outcome of such analyses often turns out to the detriment of blacks.

IMPLICATIONS

Psychology in South Africa has been conservative in that it has operated primarily within the individualistic paradigm, has adopted a mainly Eurocentric theory of human reality and has focused on adapting people to their environment. It is unlikely that Eurocentric theories of human behavior can be fully relevant for people still concerned with bread-and-butter issues in a severely oppressive society. Because of this mismatch between Western psychology and a Third World environment, psychological theory and practice in South Africa may be said to reflect the therapist's encapsulation in the bourgeois ideology, and consequently, his or her alienation from the majority of working-class clients. Accordingly, it is imperative that therapists learn about the culture and values of prospective clients since South Africa is truly a multicultural society. It is incumbent upon helping professionals to gain knowledge, awareness and skills for helping across cultures and to be sensitized to discrepancies in world-views and their impact on the therapeutic relationship, process and outcome.

In South Africa cross-cultural competencies are of major significance for facilitating a meaningful therapeutic encounter, as well as the subsequent relevant delivery of psychological services. A skilled practitioner has the awareness, knowledge and skills to intervene successfully in the lives of clients from culturally different backgrounds. Such a professional also uses strategies and techniques that are consistent with the life experiences and cultural values of clients. In order to implement these strategies and techniques, professionals must have awareness and knowledge related to issues of cultural diversity. The promise of multicultural counseling in the new South Africa is that of a new type of helping professional—the culturally skilled counselor.

CONCLUSION

The influence of the social environment and the functioning of social institutions have been influential aspects of human behavior in South Africa. Psychological approaches that are Eurocentric have been found to be largely irrelevant to the nature and needs of the majority population. The need to include indigenous healing approaches and helping approaches that incorporate spiritual dimensions is apparent, as well as the need to incorporate a community psychology approach. The present paradigm of Eurocentric theories of human behavior is ill-fitting and mismatched with an African context. Holistic approaches that address bread-and-butter needs for the majority disadvantaged population must be adopted. The counselor's role may more closely resemble that of a social worker's role with respect to the need to locate social service supports for the client. In sum, South African psychological approaches must be placed within the larger political-social and economic context.

The structural violence attendant in South Africa and the traumatizing effect it has had on the lives of all its citizens, but particularly the black majority, must be recognized. The assault on children and adolescents' self-esteem remains a critical issue and has resulted in continuous traumatic stress disorder. The mental health system cannot ignore crises in housing, employment and education—problems presently perceived to be more basic than mental health issues. Helping professionals must address high rates of family violence, a divorce rate among the three highest in the world, high incidences of depression and tension, and a sociopolitical climate that has so pressured South Africans that a generation of maladjusted children may be the result. Suggestions for dealing with these issues are presented in chapter 13, "Options and Directions for Psychology within a Framework for Mental Health Services in South Africa."

Part II

World-View and Identity

An understanding of client world-view is described in chapter 3 and the values, life experiences, cultural identity and the world-view of four major population groups, African, Indian, Afrikaner and colored, are compared in chapters 4, 5, 6 and 7. Barriers to the helping process are identified and culture-specific intervention strategies are recommended. The authors suggest that helping professionals may benefit from insights developed by Kluckhohn's world-view model and the many ways helpers may act as cultural brokers, mediating and facilitating intercultural transactions. The chapters are helpful in identifying client issues that may be associated with ethnicity. In order to meet the mental health needs of clients with differing cultural world-views, mental health professionals must be aware of such factors as systemic and environmental issues that influence intrapsychic conflicts, levels of acculturation, patterns of family systems, moral values, communication, the importance of incorporating natural support systems, and the linking of services with other systems such as resources within the community and indigenous healers. Therapists need to become culturally aware, to understand the basis for their own world-views and to understand and accept the legitimacy of world-views different from their own. In South Africa, an understanding of differing world-views is of major significance for facilitating a meaningful therapeutic encounter as well as for the subsequent relevant delivery of psychological services.

3

Understanding the Client's World-View

Problems (whether physical or mental) can be neither diagnosed nor treated without some understanding of the frame of reference of the person seeking help. McGoldrick, Pearce and Giordano (1982) recommend the following questions when seeking to work with culturally different clients:

1. What do they define as a problem?
2. What do they see as a solution to their problems?
3. To whom do they usually turn for help?
4. What are the typical family patterns of the group?
5. How do they handle lifecycle transitions?
6. What may be the difficulties for a therapist of a different background?

Many studies (Giordano & Giordano, 1977; Harwood, 1981) have shown that people differ in the following respects:

1. Their experience of pain
2. What they label as a symptom
3. How they communicate about their pain or symptoms
4. Their beliefs about the cause of their illness
5. Their attitudes toward helpers (doctors and therapists)
6. What treatment they desire or expect

Kluckhohn (1951) described value orientations of different dimensions and asserted that different cultural groups distinguished themselves by having particular world-views. These value orientations were as follows:

1. Time—the temporal focus of human life
2. Activity—the preferred pattern of action in interpersonal relations
3. The Relational Orientation—the preferred way of relating in groups
4. The Man-Nature Orientation—the way people relate to the natural or the supernatural environment
5. The Basic Nature of Man—the attitudes held about the innate good or evil in human behavior

Cultures were also thought to differ in relation to their world-view preferences as follows:

1. Time—emphasis on either past, present or future
2. Activity—emphasis on either doing, being, or being-in-becoming
3. Relational—emphasis on individual, collateral or lineal relationships
4. Man-Nature—emphasis on harmony with nature, mastery over nature or being subjugated to nature
5. Basic Nature of Man—emphasis on good, evil, or combination of good and evil

Cross-cultural counseling and psychotherapy literature have increasingly alluded to the importance of the clients' world-view. Mismatches between the counselor's and the client's ways of viewing the world, and the inability of either helper or person helped to be aware of these discrepancies, probably account for much of the breakdown in the helping process. Undoubtedly, world-view has important implications and has been identified as an important tool for counselor expertise (Sadlak & Ibrahim, 1986).

WORLD-VIEW

Individual World-View

The way in which people perceive their relationships to nature, institutions, other people and things, is referred to as world-view. Sarason (1984) proposes that we are as much possessed by, as we are possessed of, a world-view. He says that from birth onward we absorb a view of ourselves and the world in ways that are direct and indirect, purposeful and unwitting. Gregory Bateson (1944) commented as follows: "the individual is endlessly simplifying, organizing and generalizing his own view of his environment, he constantly imposes on this environment his own constructions and meanings, and these constructions and meanings are characteristic of one culture, as over against another" (p. 723).

The deliberate choosing from alternate theories on the makeup of the world formalizes a personal world-view, and world-views are, for the reasons mentioned above, correlated with cultural background, sociopolitical history and life experiences. A world-view constitutes our psychological orientation in life and can determine how we think, behave, make decisions and define events. Interacting components of a person's world-view may include (1) race, (2) ethnicity, (3) age, (4) lifestage, (5) gender, (6) lifestyle, (7) social class, (8) degree of acculturation, (9) education, (10) ordinal position in family, (11) marital status and (12) geographical locale.

Individuals must be aware of cultural complexity and of differences and similarities of practices across different cultures. In one sense culture may be seen as located both within an individual (i.e., "subjective" and internalized), as well as residing to a certain degree within a group. There may be aspects of one's own culture that may even be outside conscious awareness. The similar features of diverse cultures are evident in their constancy of a general cultural disposition and with respect to the inclusion of social system variables (age, socioeconomic status, education level, etc.). Cultures can be experienced very differently, however, with respect to contrasting value orientations and perspectives. From this perspective, each individual can be cognizant of the universality and common feel of every culture while simultaneously feeling disturbed due to variations between it and the individual's own cultural perspective.

THREE WORLD-VIEW PARADIGMS IN PSYCHOTHERAPY

Almost every counseling and psychotherapy paradigm has a world-view or cosmological foundation in which causes and effects, human behavior and psychopathology are defined, explained and predicted. Three paradigms have predominated in Western psychology: psychoanalysis, behaviorism and humanism. Psychoanalysis views human behavior in the light of unconscious factors and motivations and biological and instinctual needs, as well as psychosexual events occurring in the first five years of life. In contrast, behaviorism looks at the world from a stimulus-response foundation and contends that an understanding of the dynamics of reinforcement contingencies is needed to explain most of human behavior. Finally, humanistic psychology is a reaction to the determinism of psychoanalysis and the mechanistic impersonality of behaviorism and asserts that human behavior is a function of conscious personal and interpersonal free choice and commitment. These three ways of viewing humans in the world have been criticized for not adequately describing individuals who fall beyond the Western, white, middle-class, Anglo-American framework. For example, Diaz-Guerrero (1977) criticized these three paradigms for their focus on the self, since in many societies the family, state or society is considered the psychosocial unit, and not the individual.

Vontress (1979, 1983) subsumes these three psychotherapy world-views in his macrocosmic approach to counseling, which is based on Binswanger's (1962, 1963) three concepts: *eigenwelt*, which refers to the person's private world; *umwelt*, which refers to the physical environment; and *mitwelt*, which refers to the world of interpersonal relations. The triadic view of existence, which concentrates on the commonalities of human experience, is proposed as an appropriate paradigm for cross-cultural counseling. However, the view is criticized for excluding *welt*, the supernatural motif that underlies African epistemology and cosmology, since Africans generally believe in supernatural and ancestral causes influencing human existence. Dawis (1978) appears to adopt a behavioristic view of the world when he suggests that a useful paradigm in cross-cultural counseling might just lie in the knowledge of culture specific reinforcers (p. 466).

Alternatively, Sue (1978) presented a paradigm composed of the psychological dimension "locus of control" at one end of the continuum and "locus of responsibility" at the other end. From this perspective he describes four different kinds of world-views to be used in counseling culturally different clients. The two psychological orientations, locus of control (personal control) and locus of responsibility, are independent of one another. Clients may adopt one of four positions:

1. Internal locus of control—internal locus of responsibility (IC-IR)
2. External locus of control—internal locus of responsibility (EC-IR)
3. Internal locus of control—external locus of responsibility (IC-ER)
4. External locus of control—external locus of responsibility (EC-ER)

Each position represents a different world-view or orientation of life and members of various ethnic and racial groups, because of cultural and societal influences, have adopted different positions. If attitudes toward locus of control and locus of responsibility are known, assumptions by the therapist can be made about client motivation, self-perception and perception of the world, as well as the psychological dynamics within the therapeutic encounter.

In addition to the dimensions of locus of control and locus of responsibility, a bona fide world-view is also believed to include thoughtful answers to basic issues such as the existence and character of God, the nature of the universe and humankind, the issue of death and dying, the basis of ethics and morality and an explanation for the meaning of human history. Smith (1980) asserts that it is possible to identify the tenets of any given world-view as basically theistic, deistic, agnostic or atheistic.

SIGNIFICANCE OF CLIENT WORLD-VIEW

Cross-cultural counseling and psychotherapy literature have increasingly alluded to the importance of clients' world-view. For instance, communication is likely to be clear when counselors and clients share similar world-views. An understanding of people's structure of reasoning processes emerges from a world-view, and breakdowns in communication may be a result of differences in structure of reasoning. When world-views differ, counselors tend to attribute negative judgments to their clients. Moreover, mismatches between the counselor's and the client's ways of viewing the world, and the inability of either helper or person helped to be aware of these discrepancies, probably accounts for much of the breakdown in the helping process. It therefore follows that counselors who tend to respond according to their own conditioned values, assumptions and perspectives of reality, with total disregard for differences in world-view, may be engaging in a form of cultural oppression.

Ivey (1977) recommends that the therapist become a functional integrator who integrates positive aspects of each world-view without losing a sense of his or her own integrity. Ahia's (1984) assumption is that differences in world-view are integral to humanity, and that a more practical solution to attempting to integrate these world-views may be to retool, contextualize or culturalize psychology to new and different environments. Thus, psychologies should be modified for different people. In addition, therapists are urged to be aware of the special cultural roots of their language, and how they view their world through the unique language of their theories. Finally, as Smith (1980) notes:

> The authentic counselor, regardless of the world view identification, possesses a wholesome appreciation for both his or her values and those of the client. This authenticity allows the counselor to be personally and objectively involved in the counseling process without threatening the client's freedom, rights and integrity. (P. 587)

Authentic counselors can thus work with others in a climate of respect for world-views that differ from their own. Undoubtedly, world-view has important implications for cross-cultural counseling and psychotherapy and has been identified as an important tool for counselor expertise.

CONCLUSION

In South Africa the dominant white minority has subscribed to a Eurocentric world-view, whereas the majority population reflects an Afrocentric world-view. The Eurocentric world-view espoused by the governing white minority has mainly stressed materialism, competition, self-interest, independence and assertion, organized religion (Christianity) and a tendency to make comparative judgments (i.e., "white" supremacy). The primacy of the individual over the group has also been stressed. Consequently, whites in South Africa have emphasized a material ontology, with the highest value being placed on the acquisition of objects. Identity and self-worth are based on external criteria such as what one owns and on status symbols. Individuality, privacy and separateness are also valued. Presently, the white population in South Africa is also experiencing fear and anxiety with respect to the sweeping social changes now taking place.

An Afrocentric world-view, in contrast, has stressed a group ethic and the collective good, the unity of the universe and the notion that spirit and matter are one. A deep spirituality, which recognizes the influence of the spirit world and the ancestors on one's present behavior, is also acknowledged. Within the African life experience there may also be issues of locus of control and responsibility, both of which may be external due to the conditioning that has taken place by living in a highly authoritarian and oppressive society. A fatalistic approach to life and feelings of powerlessness may be present. Because Africans have been viewed by the dominant white culture as deficient or defective they may view themselves as helpless. Frequently they have experienced within-group or black-on-black violence as well. Violence itself may be perceived as a stress reaction to the systemic oppression and the result of being located within an inhumane culture.

What individuals see depends on whether or not it supports their view of reality, which to a large extent is culturally bound. To understand a cultural frame of reference there must be a holistic view of one's culture. Rather than trying to displace traditional theories of counseling that are based on three different world-views—psychoanalytic, humanistic and cognitive-behavioral—multicultural approaches should complement them. Counseling theories must be adapted to fit cultural perspectives.

It is a reality that the majority African population has developed personality patterns in response to white racism and oppression. In some instances there have been self as well as group deprecating behaviors, with certain members even affiliating or showing appreciation for the white minority oppressors. This can only reflect a degree of racial self-hatred toward one's own reference group. In other instances there has been ethnocentrism directed toward groups other than one's own, with some groups even rewarding criminal behavior toward these groups. These personal constructs, consequently, affect the actions of individuals. The humanistic approach can have value if used as the basis for self-awareness. Issues of self-estrangement and victimization and how they impact on all aspects of human relationships can be explored. The psychodynamic perspective could have value if it is used to emphasize the personal historical perspective of South African cultural dynamics for the individual and to identify internal states that explain the meaning of South African culture for and to the client. There may also be unconscious patterns and habits of culturally learned assumptions operating in the individual's life. The behavioral perspective can be used to link behavior change to the environment. For example, the problem of group pressure versus individual autonomy can be dealt with from this perspective. In employing either the behavioral, humanistic or psychoanalytic approach, what is important to realize is that each approach can make a contribution from its perspective if contextualized within the framework of South African society.

The following chapters present four different world-views: African, Indian, Afrikaner and colored. Mental health issues and counseling concerns relative to each world-view are also presented.

4

Beginning Life as an African Child

Africans are very conscious of their culture. Most African children receive a thorough initiation into the realm of spiritual and social traditions and values. A thorough grounding in the history of their people and their ancestors is given as well.

To comprehend African children and appreciate their behavior, counselors and educators need to understand the African value system and norms. First, it must be realized that southern Africa is not a melting pot, but instead a rich mosaic of numerous African multicultural communities—Tswana, Zulu, Sotho, Xhosa and other Pedi, Ndebele, Shangaan, Venda, Swazi, among others. For many Africans, cultural assimilation has not taken place and the practices of tribal societies prevail. Although there are diversities among African people, there are common elements as well. The African ethos is distinct from that of prevailing white society in that a common guiding set of beliefs, which have common features, exist for most Africans despite tribal affiliation. In this Afrocentric world-view there appears to be a coherent system of thought that is implicit in customs and ritual acts. Some of the major features of this system are found in attitudes toward nature, communal practices, the perception of time, the oral tradition, family customs, spiritual values and healing traditions.

HARMONY WITH NATURE

A major non-African belief is that of Manifest Destiny, a belief by a society that it has been ordained by God to conquer and rule the universe. Anglo-Americans have held this viewpoint and have sought to eradicate disease, explore space and forever conquer new frontiers. This viewpoint has also been represented graphically by the Afrikaner, who also sought to control the universe and who dominated the lives and destinies of the African majority toward this end. In contrast, the goal of the African tribe as a collective unit has been that of blending harmoniously into the flow of the universe. Acceptance of the natural order is valued, for the African sees himself/herself as part of an unbroken chain composed of all life—plant, animal, man (Busia, 1963; Holdstock, 1979).

Reverence for the earth and a desire to keep the land fertile and friendly are demonstrated in a number of rites and in labor, prayers, songs and dancing, as well as in communication with the ancestors. The African thus views the cosmos respectfully and with a sense of awe. The beauty of Africa is celebrated in poetry that eulogizes the mountains and plains, forest and desert and the great inland seas. The mystery of the universe is acknowledged. Rather than trying to control and subjugate nature, it is with humility that the African believes that nature has power that must be revered as well as used for man's good. Consequently, Africans have been able to utilize elements of their natural environment and this is reflected in their use of herbs for indigenous healing purposes.

Africans adopt a holistic approach and believe they are one with nature. Humanity is an inseparable part of the universe and man's unity with nature is stressed in African life through day-to-day activities, in human relations, in various rites and rituals and in attitudes toward work, play, love and death. Every aspect of the world is believed to be functionally related. Man is but a seed in the vast universe and the universe is replicated in each and every individual.

COMMUNAL PRACTICES

In Western thought the central facet of objective reality is the person. Emphasis is placed on self-awareness, self-fulfillment and the development of individual potential. A Western world-view thus emphasizes individuality, uniqueness and separateness as well as individual rights. In contrast, in African society the group, rather than the individual, is given paramount importance. The group really represents an extended self in that the rationale for individual existence is to insure the survival of the group. What is good for the group is thought to be good for the individual. "Individualism" is realized in group prosperity. A collective responsibility as well as commonality and a sense of peoplehood are felt. Individual rights are deemphasized and a group ethic prevails.

The African view of man in society lays more emphasis on his/her membership within a group than on the member's individuality. Group membership continues even after death and into the life beyond. Consequently, the role of ancestors, who are regarded as the living dead, takes on rich meaning. The dead, the living and the yet unborn all belong to one common family. Communal bonds are expressed in various initiation rituals and ceremonies.

Africans have a very strong sense of community, communal existence and collective responsibility. They see themselves as one with family, tribe and community and they do not regard themselves primarily as individuals. For this reason their societies are socialist in character. As Khoapa (1980) notes:

> The African sees all men as brethren; thus he is universally charitable. Africans have a strong sense of "what is mine is thine." It is held to be a moral evil to deny hospitality even to a stranger. When people travel they stop anywhere for the night and receive hospitality in that homestead. (P. 56)

Within the African value system a sense of community is a prime value. One's humanity is expressed in belonging to the whole community. It is to the whole community or tribe that total allegiance is given, for this is where one's whole existence was shaped and formed. Accordingly, there is one phenomenon reality—a communal phenomenology.

Kinship ties permeate all aspects of African life and dictate interdependence and cooperation. Individuals are closely bound to one another and nothing exists apart from the whole. In contrast to the Anglo-American frame of reference that emphasizes individualism, competition and achievement, African values stress cooperation, a "weness" ethic and tribal cohesiveness. The individual's survival is thought to be tied to the group's survival. Because of this group ethic, many acts of unselfishness, self-sacrifice and valor may be demonstrated by the individual out of love and respect for the many compatriots.

Due to the social contract existing in African societies, which lays value on behavior that contributes to the collective good, social conduct is prized that contributes to peace and equilibrium within the community. When interpersonal conflict does arise, all members affected by the conflict may participate in the conflict-resolution process. Because most African moral values emphasize social conduct and the need for interdependence, few Africans experience the sense of alienation that is common in Western society with its emphasis on individual, competitive behavior.

TIME

In the African context time is measured by events, as opposed to numerical units. Time is not a mathematically precise event, but rather an experiential happening. Unlike the Westerner, Africans are not time-bound and they do not live their lives by the clock. The future is made up of the extended present and the present is valued because it is real, tangible and can be felt and touched. The future, in contrast, cannot be guaranteed and is therefore "uncertain," and ill-defined. Life is to be lived in the present, guided by past events and memories (Busia, 1963).

For the African, time exists against the backdrop of past generations. In African thought the dead must be included with the living, since the ancestors, the "living dead," are thought to possess personal or spiritual powers that can be used for or against the living. Ancestors explain and interpret man's destiny. In a world charged with meanings, they are able to serve as a conduit and mediator. Ancestors are thought to be intermediaries between God and men and to possess the secrets of the universe. Africans believe that many of their departed kin keep constant watch over the living in order to ensure that they observe moral laws. The past is greatly valued since ancestors play a vital spiritual role in the lives of those in most African societies (Buhrmann, 1977; Khoapa, 1980).

In African society, the direction of one's life is from the present dimension backward into the past. Time itself is very elastic, and the event occurs when one gets there, regardless of the time it has been scheduled. Time is conceived of as a phenomenon and not as measured by clocks and calendars. Time is flexible, not precise (Mbiti, 1970). In the South African context it may be conjectured that along with the present and the past, the future is also becoming of increasing value because of changing socioeconomic and political conditions and the strength of the liberation movement.

SPIRITUAL VALUES

One of the great difficulties in studying African religion and philosophy is that there are no sacred scriptures or texts, due to the prevailing oral tradition. However, religious beliefs and practices can be found throughout African societies. Spirituality is such an integral part of the African's existence that it and he/she are inseparable. Gbekobow (1984) noted that the "daily life of an African child is a continuous initiation into the realm of spiritual and social fundamentals of the community" (p. 228).

Beliefs are corporate and religious acts are communal. Faith is woven into the full pattern of life and God is a presence of an infinite and eternal energy from which all things proceed. There is a perception of a personal being and a notion that there is an all pervasive "energy" that is the source, sustainer and essence of all phenomena.

Because of the love of nature, natural temples are water, earth, air and fire, and worship is often outdoors on the banks of rivers. Unlike its Western counterparts, traditional religion in Africa is not proselytized but is simply woven into the fabric of daily life. Presently Christianity has undergone a numerical expansion, and surprisingly, Africans do not view Christianity as a white, imported religion. Protestant churches have largely remained "Western," and traditional, rather than indigenous. Hymns and sermon texts, in the main, have not been Africanized.

God is viewed as a force shrouded in mystery and dreams are believed to be a major vehicle by which God communicates with man. God is also believed to be omnipotent and charged with power that can be either beneficial or dangerous to man. In the realm between God and man are thought to lie many powers and principalities, both good and bad. This fact accounts for many of the strange and mysterious happenings in the world, which can be explained as being the work of either spirits, magical forces or witches and demons. The ancestors are also thought to possess power over the living and to control the people's destiny. They are thought to possess supernatural powers and to be intermediaries between God and man. Supplications and special offerings to the ancestors on man's behalf may be made (Zahran, 1979).

Africans hold a deep spirituality and exercise their belief in a supernatural power through a variety of acts woven into the fabric of daily life. The religious forms may be manifested through faith healing, diviners who decipher messages intended for man, and charismatic modes such as speaking in tongues. Diviners also clarify various situations that may occur in the lives of many Africans and give advice on the choice of marriage partners, vocational guidance and suggestions on travel plans (Buhrmann, 1977).

The spiritual dimension in the lives of Africans is inseparable from their daily life and activities. Praise to the supreme being is evident in song, dance, poetry, prayers and rituals (Khoapa, 1980).

ROLE OF THE ORAL TRADITION AND THE ARTS

Although there are no sacred texts, Africans have used different methods of recording and preserving their rich heritage. Important messages and information are transmitted orally and it has been through the oral transmission of African fables, proverbs and legends that adults have communicated values to the youth. Within many tribes there is even a designated oral historian who serves as a link between the past and present. Beliefs and traditions have been orally handed down generation after generation. Such a tradition of "oral preservation" places tremendous importance on the function of memory. The legacy of African retention is illustrated in a modern example of today's mainstream "rap" music.

Features of the oral tradition also include a high degree of vocal participation by those present and a response to what is being said. This is known as the call-response (Smith, 1974). Another feature is that of the praise reciter who will orally recite praise poems and tales of bravery and achievement by great warriors of the tribe. Poetry of nature, folk stories and proverbs are also related orally as well as worship literature.

The oral system may also be combined with dance, music, song and iconographic art. It is often through dance that the history of a people is enacted. As with the oral tradition, dance is woven into the fabric of community life. It is often a spontaneous emanation to an event and is never detached from the lives of African people. Events that could be celebrated through dance may be the installation of a chief, the birth of a baby, the onset of puberty, a marriage, harvesting a good crop or even resolution of a dispute. Dancing may be done as either an appeal or as thanksgiving for rain, sun, children, marriage and the like.

Because the African is close to nature, dancing often emulates the rhythm and movement of birds, animals, trees, waves in the ocean or other features of the living environment. Intense affective involvement is conveyed through dance and all of the emotions of love, hatred, fear, joy, sorrow, disgust and amazement may be expressed through body movement. The drum is often used and chants and songs accompany the rhythmic movement. African dance is also usually a collective act with a great deal of participation. The legacy and importance of dance is treasured, for priests, warriors, hunters and healers were primarily dancers.

Creativity is a strong characteristic of an African society and the arts are an integral part of a way of life. Music also plays a vital role in the lives of Africans. Improvisation is often the rule and African music combines song and dance. Music often depicts the daily tasks and routines as well as major events and happenings. It is also used to reflect on these experiences and can be the voice of the tribe and communal sentiment. Music often transmits tribal knowledge and can also mark various rites and ceremonies. Many songs are choral with each improvisation being a new group creation.

It is through singing that tribal bonding is accomplished and corporate feelings strengthened (Mbiti, 1970). Music transmits the history of the people and their culture and is also used to resolve conflict. Music also enacts the various life situations and rituals. In truth, however, the primary purpose of music is to preserve the oral tradition (Burlen, 1930).

Other art forms are adornment, through dress and jewelry, and the wearing of bright, harmonious colors. Basket weaving, wood carving and beadwork represent additional art forms (Thompson, 1974).

FAMILY VALUES

Apartheid in South Africa has impacted negatively on family relations. The African family has developed variegated forms according to the different situations it has encountered. These variations may be matriarchal in character whereby African males are marginal and ineffectual figures in the family constellation. The strength of the family has been undermined by the impact of influx control (a government policy that set out to limit the urbanization of Africans by restricting them to residence in tribal areas and resulting in an overall migrant labor pattern) and by the process of urbanization. The African family as an institution of society has thus been fragmented due not only to influx control laws, but also by the creation of Bantustans (resettlement reserves for blacks), urbanization, and rural living conditions and demands. Due to these factors, parental separation occurs and parents are often unable to meet the child's needs and developmental demands. Many times the major responsibility for child rearing has come to rest on the mother. The absence of male role models for protracted periods of time and lack of preparation for future parenthood all too often have become the norm for African children (Burman & Reynolds, 1986).

The employment of African women in domestic service in white households is a major feature of the economic structure of South Africa. In 1985 approximately 76 percent of white families had at least one domestic (Goodwin, 1985). Economic necessity propels many African women into the labor market, although reluctantly. For example, in a national sample of African working women (Cock, Emdon & Klugman, 1986), the vast majority were mothers as well as workers;

over 96 percent had children, over half of whom were preschoolers. In leaving their children at home, many female African workers have no available family members to take care of their children and may use forms of childcare outside their own family such as neighbors and childminders. A report on daycare published in 1983 found that of a preschool population of over 4 million African children, only 37 percent were looked after in day-care facilities and nurseries (Reilly & Hofmeyr, 1983). Because of the legacy of apartheid, there exists a pressing need to provide social services and supportive care for African children.

The bearing of children is an obligation in African societies and that obligation is seen as a way of ensuring more labor and therefore a more productive group. Few concepts are as deeply ingrained in the African psyche as the need and the desire to reproduce. In many tribes an infertile man is ostracized and a barren woman shunned. Parents may arrange marriages, and there is great respect for and confidence in the wisdom and age of African parents. Marriage of one man to two or more women is an accepted tribal practice and in agricultural societies ensures even more labor. Because the producing of children is a high value, sexual roles are clearly defined and parents do not allow children to confuse their sexual identity. However, gender roles are flexible in that males may be involved in a variety of "female" tasks such as cooking and cleaning without putting their male prowess at risk.

In most African cultures children assume responsibility at a very early stage, even before the age of three. From the start they are considered to be producers, not consumers. Disasa (1988) comments:

> In Africa, traditional education prepares the children for life providing them with ways of actually practicing life through a learning-by-doing method. Learning is combined with ongoing responsibilities ranging from relatively simple jobs to more difficult tasks. Running errands and guarding the home during the day while parents are away are among the simple tasks. More rigorous tasks include tilling and cultivating plots of land, tending domestic animals all day long, drawing water from a river and well and collecting firewood for use. Going to formal school for those who are fortunate enough to live within a school vicinity or district means additional responsibility. (P. 18)

Boating (1983) asserts that there is a harmonious transition from youth obligations to adult responsibilities in African tradition:

> To a large extent there was no conflict between what children were expected to do and what was happening in their environment, what was real was not different from what was taught. Consequently, children's acceptance and appreciation of the morals and norms of their society facilitated communication between them and adults . . . in a nutshell, customs and examples were heavily relied upon as the principle educational agents. (P. 335)

The role of the family is that of moral education, and from the beginning African children are instructed to aspire to a good reputation. Children respect adults and adults respect other adults. Hierarchy based on age is greatly respected and older persons are thought to have wisdom. In African society, however, females are not given equality with males and a patriarchal value system operates with males presumed to have more value than females. Nduka (1980) summarized the values of traditional societies in Africa as handed down by the family, as follows: "respect for human dignity, sense of community, mutual aid, hospitality, respect for legitimate and humane authority, courage and gallantry, and respect for authentic African moral and religious values" (p. 159).

In South Africa, African children have learned endurance and perseverance early in their lives. Due to the harshness and injustice of apartheid, the pain of hunger, lack of adequate clothing, difficulty encountered while walking long distances and lack of basic educational opportunities and materials are among the greatest obstacles they face. The African child has thus learned to develop early maturity in self-discipline, great patience and a willingness and determination to endure hardships.

INDIGENOUS HEALING PRACTICES

Kleinman (1980), a psychiatrist trained in anthropology, concluded that:

> In the same sense in which we speak of religion or language or kinship or cultural system we can view medicine as a cultural system, a language of symbolic meaning anchored in particular arrangement of social institutions and patterns of interpersonal interactions. In every culture illness, the response to it, the individuals experiencing it and treating it, and the social relationships relating to it are all systematically interrelated. . . . These include patterns of belief about the causes of illness, norms governing choice and evaluation of treatment, socially legitimated statuses, roles, power relationships, interaction settings and institutions. . . . Patients and healers are basic components of such systems and thus healers are embedded in specific configurations of cultural meanings and social relationships. They cannot be understood apart from this context. (Pp. 24–25)

Accordingly, the ways in which sick people are responded to by family and practitioners are all aspects of social reality in African culture and behavioral norms are all cultural constructions.

In South Africa there have been numerous traditional healers. Such practitioners of indigenous healing included sangomas, sorcerers, herbalists, diviners and faith healers. With respect to the mental health needs of the majority population, these practitioners represent a neglected potential that can be tapped since indigenous healing is woven into the fabric of community life (Buhrmann, 1977). In the eyes of the African, the healers carry the messages intended for humanity and the society in which he or she lives. Such healers are thought to be a conduit for the messages of the cosmos and are believed to possess the skill of penetrating and imparting the secrets of the universe. The healer is thus viewed as a mediator between the world and human beings.

With respect to treatment strategies, Western medicine divides illness into the different categories of somatic, psychological and psychosomatic. African people, in contrast, adopt a holistic approach. They say, "When part of me is ill, all of me is ill." The use of traditional healing involves the whole person and uses the social, psychological and spiritual as well as the physical domain. Dancing, singing, rituals and ceremonies are used by the healer. By giving external and concrete form to anxieties through the use of rituals, threatening images can be ventilated and thereby become meaningful and less ominous. Traditional healing is also advantageous to the mental health system because it not only involves curative intervention but is used in relation to the prevention of illness or misfortune as well. The indigenous healer, who is viewed as psychologist, physician, priest and prophet by many in an African society, has an established credibility and is a pervasive influence in the lives of the majority of peoples in developing societies in Africa (Green, 1988).

The healer is thus a full part of the sociocultural life of the members of the community as a whole. In the use of such healers there is community participation in treatment and there is a perfect match between healing communities and Africa's communal system. In sum, traditional healers can make a valuable contribution to mental health prevention and treatment.

MENTAL HEALTH ISSUES AND COUNSELING APPROACHES

There are significant differences between African world-view and Western psychologies. Western theories such as psychoanalysis, humanistic (Rogers, Gestalt, existential) and cognitive-behavioral (rational-emotive, reality therapy, Beck) either/or stress the individual, achievement motivation, the scientific method, rationality and direct self-disclosure. Most of the mental health models that have been used have been derived from British and American models where institutions and lifestyles are relatively similar. Traditional models of intervention have represented both a limiting and oppressive mode, particularly with African clients who have suffered the inequities of the South African racist system. Consequently, it is difficult if not impossible to understand African people using traditional theories developed by white psychologists to explain white behavior. Adaptation of existing psychological models to the African world-view and the reality of the African perspective demands that the construction of counseling theories take into account the factors of cultural identity and the social and political realities involved in existing symbiotically with the dominant white culture.

One very real issue is that Africans in South Africa have been systematically persecuted and exploited as a group. An African who is not suspicious of whites is denying certain objective and basic realities of the African experience in South Africa. Non-African counselors, psychologists, social workers, guidance personnel and educators are going to have to learn to work constructively with this hostility. Many Africans may not feel comfortable talking with whites and may feel too angry with them to be able to focus on anything else. If white helpers are able to drop their own defensiveness about being labelled "the enemy" and acknowledge the legitimacy of the African point of view, there most probably could be movement toward a more cooperative relationship. However, white helpers must also be prepared for rejection in some instances.

A second counseling issue is that of low self-image. Most Africans have been psychologically crippled to a greater or lesser degree by the effects of apartheid. The results of being oppressed and victimized may be translated into self-loathing, a confused self-identity and low achievement. In South Africa, Africans have too long depended on white society for a definition of self and have too long had adaptive patterns of Anglo-American ways superimposed on them. For too long a "deficit personality paradigm" has been promoted by a white ruling government. Behind the mask of compliance and subservience often is repressed rage and a burning desire for self-definition. A major mental health goal that will contribute toward healthy psychological functioning for Africans is that of heightened self-esteem and self-reclamation, for example, an Afrocentric identity. For many Africans there currently exists an alien self or an antiself. Therefore, long after apartheid, the African's journey will continue to embrace the search for identity and self-reclamation.

A third counseling issue is that of the methods employed in helping African clients. African children and adolescents need tools for dealing with their problems. The notion of sedentary talk as a medium for client-counselor interaction should be challenged. "Just listening" is not enough and counseling approaches need to accommodate modeling, simulations, contracts and skills for dealing with the environment. Particular approaches that could help are those dealing with conflict resolution, coping skills, problem-solving strategies and vocational planning. Because of the emotional scarring of apartheid, strategies to engender feelings of empowerment would also be helpful.

Techniques and approaches also must be based on African culture. Art forms such as poetry, dance, music and songs and storytelling should be incorporated. The importance of the oral tradition and the love and respect for tradition should be acknowledged. Bringing in the client's extended support system and kin would be helpful, as well as acknowledging the roles that both indigenous healers and the ancestors could play in problem solving.

A fourth counseling issue is that of expectations. An African client will expect the counselor to be more directive and structured and to behave more like a "doctor," for example, diagnosing and describing. Interventions that assume an equalitarian relationship and a permissive ambiguous structure will more than likely fail. Advice seeking would be a goal for the African client and the therapist would be expected to act like an authority figure.

Another issue is the importance of nonverbal communication. African gestures, body movements and nuances must be understood. The counselor placing emphasis on verbally expressed feelings is likely not to perceive the real nonverbal message. It must also be realized that the counselor cannot make an assumption of trying to elicit full and direct self-disclosure. Being able to keep a secret is prized in an African culture and one does not tell shameful things about the family to outsiders. The skilled counselor will be able to "read" nonverbal behavior, for it may signify the African client's discomfort, embarrassment and so on. In a society where Africans have not been allowed to speak out freely, movement and gesture are extremely important and constitute the real message.

In general, Africans know no such thing as "personal physical space" and have a great deal of physical contact while carrying on a conversation. There is a much shorter distance between persons than one would find with Anglo-Americans. In addition to the variable of a shorter personal space, variables regarding eye contact must also be acknowledged. Direct eye contact will be regarded as a sign of rudeness, and the Western tradition of looking at the person and nodding your head is not necessary. More peripheral vision will be used by the African client. For the counselor to assume that the African client is being inattentive, shy or bored is a false assumption. Additionally, the Western conversation convention of client self-disclosure and maximum volume of speech may not be valid. Instead, silence on the part of the African client may indicate a respect for the helper rather than an unwillingness to continue. Additionally, Africans relate to one another spontaneously rather than following a protocol and formal conventions. A formal counseling setting could be off-putting. How furniture in an office is arranged, where the seats are located and where you seat the client may have meanings and implications that enhance or retard the counseling relationship.

Counseling approaches also need to be holistic and to recognize the effects of environmental deprivation. Because many African households are characterized by crowding, these conditions create stress factors and offer poor learning conditions. Poverty places many African children at risk and it is doubtful that children who are hungry can be optimally helped in the counseling encounter. In the new South Africa the counselor's role will probably more closely resemble that of a social worker in that he or she will need to locate resources and make referrals.

It should also be remembered that because of the struggle for survival, many Africans are here-and-now oriented. Goal setting should represent immediate, achievable goals rather than long-term strategies. Issues may typically center on the basic issues of survival and security, as clients are not inclined to see the value in a long-term counseling process. African clients may want help in getting information and finding resources to solve immediate practical concerns in their social environment. For these reasons, action-oriented approaches are more relevant than talk therapy, which solely emphasizes the exploration of feelings.

Counselors attempting to help African clients also need to know how African cultural systems view the helping relationship and how individuals within the system solve problems traditionally. From this perspective it must be remembered that for Africans, healing often takes place in environments that might seem inappropriate. There may be loud music, chanting, dancing and other activities going on simultaneously. Clients accustomed to such environments may be a bit anxious when left alone in a quiet private office with a counselor.

CONCLUSION

The following questions may also be useful to consider when employing counseling methods to help the African client:

1. Does the theory allow for the inclusion of the uniqueness of the African experience in the understanding of individual functioning?
2. Does the method used also acknowledge within group differences and acknowledge the uniqueness of the individual and the ways in which the client may differ from the mainstream African culture?
3. Do the approaches used allow the choice of goals and values that are in keeping with the African experience and that are perceived as meaningful and valuable to the African client?
4. Does the therapeutic process involve modes or behaviors that are culturally relevant to the African experience?

The counseling environment must fit the preference of the African client and it is possible that many African clients tend to prefer a structured, direct interview and one with a practical orientation, with the counselor's role being that of giving advice and suggestion. However, it is also possible that such clients may have very different preferences. In keeping with a multicultural perspective, the counselor should be adept at utilizing culture-specific techniques if the need arises, yet aware enough not to stereotype or slot African clients whose needs may be very different.

5

Born into an Indian Community

Hinduism developed on Indian soil approximately 2,500 years ago and has spread out geographically to include southeast Asia (Bali, Cambodia, Ceylon, Nepal) as well as other parts of the world (Kakar, 1971). Asian Indians first came to Natal as indentured laborers to work on sugar plantations. The first group arrived in 1860 on contracts for a period of three (later five) years after which they could become automatically free. Having secured their freedom they were able to either remain in South Africa or to secure free passage back to India. Their contracts to remain in South Africa could be renegotiated to include a further service period of five years. Most of those who came from India elected to remain. Initially, although they had been recruited as laborers on sugar plantations, they also secured employment in the railways (Ferguson-Davie, 1952).

Prior to 1860 there were virtually no Indians in South Africa. Today there are approximately 0.9 million (Wilson & Ramphele, 1989, p. 3). Of this number many follow different religions such as Hinduism, Islam, various denominations of Christianity, Zorasterianism or no religion at all. Hinduism remains the predominant religion in South Africa, with over 70 percent of the Indian population being adherents.

The Indian population in South Africa has had to cope with social discrimination and various political and legal disabilities in the same way as Africans and coloreds. There has been a long history of opposition to white rule. Gandhi, the pioneer of Indian independence, first developed techniques of nonviolent resistance to the British in South Africa, where he helped found the Natal Indian Congress before World War I (Hellman, 1949).

Because Hindus represent the dominant Indian group in South Africa, their world-view and its implications for counseling will be described. Though different in certain respects, much of their cultural conduct in urban and rural areas is directly derived from sacred Indian texts and from traditional Indian sources.

CHILD DEVELOPMENT

All families transmit a particular "version" of culture to their children. Regardless of the familial or cultural context in which children are socialized, the task of the family in this process is universal. The family's task is to interpret to their children the values, beliefs and appropriate behavioral patterns of their culture. The task for children is to acquire the cultural knowledge and skills that will enable them to participate effectively in the cultural life of the family and later in the cultural life of the larger community. In order to accomplish their task, all families within a society establish patterns of interaction and communication, customs and beliefs, and expectations of behavior and conduct.

The Hindu concept is that the personality of any particular individual extends before birth and after death, a process of identity that extends over many generations. Due to the belief in karma, certain personality and character traits are thought to be present at birth. This concept will be described more fully in a later section.

When a Hindu child is born, a period of forty days is used to keep the mother and child in close seclusion with constant bodily contact used to insure bonding. The seclusion period is also used for the purpose of purification, which is accomplished through sequestering both mother and child. Afterward, numerous associations with the outside world are formed, with the mother still intent on ministering to the child's every need. Considerable interest is shown in all activities such as feeding, crawling and walking. Frequent periods of repose are thought especially important, for a baby is believed to grow in its sleep. Waking is psychologically important, and since it is believed that the first person one sees will influence the rest of the day, a mother should be cheerful and smiling when her baby opens its eyes. The period of extreme maternal indulgence continues until the birth of a new baby. If the child remains the youngest, he or she continues to receive maternal attention and could be breast-fed for as long as three or four years (Prabhu, 1954).

There are numerous significant others who are involved in the tasks of child rearing as well. For example, bathing the baby is usually a privilege reserved for the grandmother. Protocol dictates that the mother must allow anyone in the home the pleasure of joining in the child-rearing tasks and in nurturing the child. Parents are discouraged from being possessive and are encouraged to share their blessings with others (Kakar, 1979).

Although the child receives considerable attention, restraint is taught as well. Modesty and humility are emphasized, and even in babies, nakedness is considered an embarrassment. Certain behavioral codes of dress are also enforced such as loose, nonrevealing clothing. Restraint is also encouraged in interpersonal relationships. Individual desires are sometimes suppressed in the interest of the family and from the time a child can understand, he/she is conditioned to be fair and responsible in social participation. Children are not encouraged to develop as independent individuals but as cooperative members of the family and the broader community. Contributing to society and to one's fellow beings are values inculcated from an early age (Kuper, 1958).

From childhood, instruction in correct behavior is given and various ceremonies and events reinforce appropriate behavior. Many of the tasks the child is given are socially useful ones in character development and all efforts are critically appraised. For most children there are usually few periods of free play and few chances to be irresponsible in the world of make-believe. For girls, there is instead training in speaking quietly and walking lightly and much preparation in learning to be ladylike. Boys also are indoctrinated into the rules of social etiquette. Such early conditioning may result in marked inhibition and a lack of spontaneity and even toys may be treated with extreme care as if they are household possessions.

Children usually begin to receive discipline around the age of three. Acts of foul language, property destruction and immodest behavior are all punishable offenses. The family is regarded as the primary socializing agent and held responsible for enforcing appropriate behavior. Parent-child communications are formal and proceed from parent to child. Should the child misbehave and receive discipline, he or she, when crying, is not picked up and reassured. Various family slogans are used instead that he/she "is given reason for crying" and "a child must be taught that it pays for everything it does" (Kuper, 1958, p. 125). In Indian society the promise of reward as well as the threat of punishment is used to induce socially approved behavior (Surya, 1969).

THE KINSHIP SYSTEM

The importance of kinsmen is highly valued in Hindu culture. It is from them that social values and behavior are imparted. One also develops a sense of collective responsibility from this structure. For example, the term "father" carries with it the responsibility of looking after those in the extended household. To help a kinsmen is a primary obligation and one does not look after one's own children without also showing concern for the needs of children of kin (Kakar, 1979).

Kinsmen also keep one another informed about any important matters, such as births, deaths and job changes, and communication is mainly by direct personal visits, with letter writing being rare. Social visits extending from a few days to a number of weeks are common, as well as duty visits in time of trouble (Meer, 1966).

Kinship ties are seldom if ever severed and relationships become quite intrusive because it is believed that the behavior of each individual affects the reputation of the entire system. "Privacy" is virtually nonexistent, and almost all matters are a cause for common concern. If behavior is not acceptable, such as an individual who drinks excessively or gambles, much gossiping occurs and members may even disassociate themselves in order to indicate disapproval and allow censure to serve as a deterrent.

The completely isolated individual is rare and individuals who are on their own will be incorporated as a kinsman into a family. For example, widows usually stay with relatives or may play a grandmother role in another family. A custom still held by many is that no respectable Hindu girl is allowed to live alone, as to do so indicates loose morals (Kuper, 1958).

THE EXTENDED FAMILY

The term *kutum* is used to describe the family and a kutum includes a male head, his wife, unmarried children, unmarried brothers or sisters of the male head, younger married brothers and married sons with their wives and children. The number of kutum members living at any particular time varies from a couple of individuals to over a hundred.

Structurally the kutum is conceptualized as a hierarchy, with the eldest living patriarch at the apex and constituting with his wife the highest authority. Next comes the younger married brothers and their wives, then unmarried brothers, then the patriarch's married sons and his brother's married sons and so on to the youngest generation of descendants. The kutum is not an organization of independent and equal family units, but is composed of graded subunits interacting through bonds of patrilineal descent and of marriage. Most professional men follow the pattern of bringing their wives to live with their parents for a certain period of time when they begin married life.

SEX ROLES

In traditional Indian society social relations are hierarchical. In each order the status and roles of individuals are further regulated by age and sex. With siblings of the same sex, seniority regulates relationships and particular respect is shown older brothers and sisters. The oldest brother also has the responsibility for both the education and the marriage of younger brothers. Special privileges and authority over females of their own age group are given to males. However, males must give submission to the authority of older males, as well as to senior women.

Sex role differences are further pronounced in the roles in the family. Boys are allowed freer rein while also taught that their role is to protect and look after their sisters. The brother is the guardian of his sister's morals and must insure that her companions are proper. Chaste behavior is mandatory and should an illegitimate pregnancy occur, the family will be strongly condemned and the girl married off to the nearest widower.

Whereas a male is supposed to partake of worldly experience, a female is expected to be a paragon of virtue. Her behavior and actions can bring either shame or glory to the family itself. A dual portrait is painted of women in the sacred texts, for they are shown as virtuous wives and mothers or as temptresses who are ready to strike. Because females are perceived as having the potential to exercise a dual nature, brothers frequently escort their sisters to different events, ensuring that they are safe in their company.

Puberty is regarded as a major milestone in the life of a Hindu girl, and the girl's behavior becomes even more restricted. She is watched even more closely, and there is strict supervision of activities. A great deal of attention is paid to what the neighborhood is saying about each girl, because a bad reputation can injure the possibility of a good marriage.

MARRIAGE

Romantic love is idealized in Hindu literature, but is not regarded as a good basis for marriage. Real love is thought to come after marriage, not before. The ideals of marital conduct are symbolically portrayed in the stylized marriage vows. A variety of symbolic acts bind the couple together, such as the knotting of the groom's sash to the end of the bride's sari and the exchange of garlands. The authority the husband has over his wife is demonstrated when bride and groom circle the fire, with the bride leading the first few rounds and then yielding the lead to her husband.

The Hindu wife is subservient to her husband and is valued for her wisdom and virtue. Chastity prior to marriage and lifelong faithfulness to her spouse are the ideal norm. Because of their natures women are considered to be more pure than men, although both are expected to strive for virtue. Marriage itself represents not only a sacred and holy bond between two people, but serves as a contract between respective kin as well.

Women are expected to assume a domestic role in caring for the home and bearing and rearing children. Wives are not supposed to work, except should economic necessity dictate or if they are specially educated workers who are trained for a profession that will benefit society (Kakar, 1979).

Should the young people elect to live in his parent's home the first few years of marriage, which is often customary, the Hindu daughter-in-law is expected to be docile and to give deference to her mother-in-law and to avoid direct and intimate contact with male in-laws. These latter relationships must take on the character of that existing between father and daughter or brother and sister, for strong religious, social and legal emphasis is placed on safeguarding the sexual rights of her husband.

Because of the strong attachment between the husband and his mother, the daughter-in-law is placed in an inferior position in his parents' home. She is acutely aware that her mother-in-law's approval is critical and that she must uncomplainingly perform domestic chores when asked. Difficult relationships also exist between the daughter-in-law and the husband's other female relatives. It is she who must adapt to their way of life and only with the passing of many years and having her own house does the Hindu wife become more removed from in-law control. The Indian household may never be completely independent, however. The wife and her husband still are expected to consult the larger extended family on matters of importance.

In Hinduism, as exemplified in the kinship system and the extended family, the basic structure of personality is relational rather than individual. The primary emphasis is on the structure of the family and kinship relations. It is through these structures that individuals relate to one another.

RELIGIO-PHILOSOPHICAL CONCEPTS

As previously described, in traditional Indian society an ideal society is hierarchical and characterized by ranked social groups into which one is born. This is known as caste, and each caste has a social function and a traditional occupation. Class structure (caste) is thought to be divinely made and not a human device. This social law is believed to be in keeping with the law of the universe. Accordingly, each person has a part to play in the social order. Caste represents a closed social system and this concept could not be transported totally by those from India into the new South African society. Additionally, in South Africa, Indians are grouped together by race in a total structure. Accordingly, the traditional caste system can only operate indirectly. Therefore, although caste is not a feature of South African Indian society, the notion that rank and hierarchy are intrinsic to human relations has been retained and is a major feature of family relations as previously described.

The classical Hindu literature of the Rg-Veda, the Upanishads and the Bhagavad-Gita have influenced Hindu traditions and customs. Four basic concepts are needed to understand this philosophy:

1. *Dharma*—codes and rules which define goodness, maturity and appropriateness of behavior
2. *Karma*—the propulsion from previous incarnation, present deed and future destiny (which has wrongly been characterized as fatalism)
3. *Maya*—the illusion of real knowledge and causes (which Westerners might describe as reality)
4. *Atman*—the person, not as an individual but as part of ultimate cosmic unity or absolute (Pedersen, 1978a)

These concepts are found in the religious literature and are concerned with the struggle between good and evil. The most striking characteristic of Indian religion is the concept of karma, the transmigration of the soul and the belief that each individual passes through many births. A constant theme in Hindu writing is that of suffering. The concept of karma posits that an individual reaps what he/she sows but also sows the seeds of his/her karma. Accordingly, the present is casually determined by the past, yet the future lies within an individual's hands inasmuch as that individual is able to initiate now the causes that will have results in the future. The concept of moksha represents the end of the endless cycle of rebirths and represents a release from ignorance and suffering. Dharma emphasizes the codes of appropriate behavior and the belief that there are various paths appropriate to different individuals that can lead to liberation: the path of work, the path of knowledge and the path of devotion.

An ancient prayer widely used in India petitions is that an individual be led from illusion to reality, from ignorance to knowledge and from mortality to immortality. Contained in this prayer are the concepts of both maya and atman. Maya denotes the search for reality and atman the realization of the ultimate nature of reality.

Hinduism represents an attempt to answer two related questions: (1) What is man, actual and ideal? and (2) How can actual man become ideal man? Maya concerns the rediscovery of the nature of the real self and the realization that the material world is false and illusory. Atman represents an awareness of one's soul as well as an awareness of Brahman (the ground of our being) and underlying reality. The aim of worship is a state of union with the absolute universal self (Brahman) (Murphy & Murphy, 1968). Hinduism thus places an emphasis on the interior life, a quest for enlightenment and a discovery of oneness with the supreme reality or the God within. Atman represents the realization of the soul's true nature.

There is also a recognition in Hinduism that people differ in their level of spiritual development. Traditionally four stages have been described which correspond to the different stages of life:

1. *Student*—must study the Hindu traditions and values, particularly expressed in the sacred literature
2. *Householder*—the task is to foster a family, undertake an occupation and perform other duties and obligations to society
3. *Forest hermit*—the individual is supposed to leave home with his wife and meditate on the realities that will bring about liberation from the world and from rebirth
4. *Wandering holy man*—the individual is to abandon everyone in order to strive for knowledge that will emancipate him for the cycles of rebirth

These four stages of development indicate a progression from self-preoccupation to time spent on uninterrupted meditation, to reflection and self-examination and last, for turning away from all earthly pursuits. In the later stages the individual begins to remove himself from society and to renounce the world.

Hinduism also believes that no right path can be found without instruction, through initiation by a qualified teacher (guru). Because individuals differ in their level of spiritual development, the training any individual needs to undergo should be adjusted to whatever stage he or she is in. The ultimate state of liberation is to be gradual rather than instantaneous. Hinduism is regarded as one of the most tolerant of all religions and is open-minded regarding one's spiritual journey and the path one takes.

Hinduism is a religion, a philosophy and a social system. It represents a life-centered philosophical, religious and ethical approach. In Hinduism the individual is deemphasized, and an emphasis is placed on the importance of social relationships. This is in direct conflict with a Western view that sees an individual as a separate entity distinct from society and culture. The Hindu system of child bearing also emphasizes continuous dependency relationships and the importance of kinship and the extended family system. Hindu culture derives its strength from the existence of a large body of sacred and traditional literature. The guru (teacher) is honored together with parents, and the value of learning is indoctrinated from childhood. Additional family values stress education and high academic and occupational achievement. The desire for success is an ethic that motivates children and encourages them to excel.

Unlike Christianity, Buddhism or Mohammedanism, Hinduism is not the one product of any single individual but a synthesis of many ideas over time. Hinduism recognizes all divine personalities as different embodiments of the same underlying reality and recognizes that there are a variety of religious paths, not one. There is great tolerance, and there is no exclusiveness and belief that only a few individuals are on the right path.

Accordingly, Hinduism is not a narrow formal religion but rather an approach to life that has developed over many thousands of years and has synthesized many different ideas and practices. Hinduism represents a tension which exists between two demands that must be harmonized: (1) that a human being is a social animal governed by physical needs and who must live with other humans and (2) that an individual is also a uniquely spiritual and solitary animal who yearns to transcend all physical and social limitations.

HEALING TRADITIONS

Psychological distress and disorders are explained within a religious framework in terms of either spirit possession or violation of some religious or moral principle. Healing may take the form of an appeal to a supernatural power or through prescribing right conduct and belief.

Kakar (1971) classified the healing traditions of India into three categories: (1) local and folk traditions, (2) mystical traditions and (3) medical traditions. In local traditions psychological disorders are generally attributed to possession by a spirit. In the second healing tradition, mysticism, religious leaders may use prayer meetings or private audiences with individuals who need help, using song and chants as well as devotional passages. Yogi exercises and other forms of meditation may also be used. In the third form, the indigenous medical tradition tries to achieve cohesiveness between the body and mind and to take a holistic view of illness. Any illness whether physical or psychological is viewed in its total context. Psychological practices such as meditation may be used, but physical treatment procedures are also used along the same lines as the general treatment of physical disorders.

COUNSELING IMPLICATIONS

First of all, in counseling, the Indian client may be reluctant to exhibit openness because restraint is viewed as a sign of maturity in Hindu culture. Revelation of personal problems is thought to reflect negatively on the whole family. To admit difficulties may be to arouse feelings of having failed the family. For this reason a better focus at the outset would be on educational, vocational and other concrete problems rather than on social or emotional concerns.

Additionally, the unstructured counseling session in which the client is expected to do most of the talking will be stressful. Hindu clients come to the counseling session with the expectation of a hierarchical relationship and with the notion that the counselor will function as a guide and teacher (guru). It is anticipated that sessions will be structured and roles clearly defined rather than be permissive and ambiguous. The Hindu client will expect advice to flow down from the authority figure. The client role is thus perceived as one of receiving guidance and instruction from the guru silently and respectfully. There may be the feeling of intense discomfort if the counselor tries to engage the client in a mutual democratic dyad relationship.

The Hindu client's world-view must also be accepted and he/she encouraged to make choices that are appropriate to perceived cultural reality. Counseling approaches must accommodate the Hindu meditative and contemplative approach and its emphasis on the interior life. Humanistic approaches that emphasize exploration would represent goodness of fit. Such approaches would also represent a value position on individual responsibility, for Hindus believe that no one is ever the cause of either the fortune or misfortune of another and that the individual alone is the cause of his/her life and its events. In Hindu terms no person can solve another's problems, for each must work out his/her own salvation.

Rogerian approaches would also be fitting in their view that man is in the process of becoming. Hindus believe in the process of development and of evolving perfection. Hinduism is a process, not a result, a process of the perfecting man. Rogers discussed the self one truly is, movement toward trust of self and the directions toward the true self. The drawback of the Rogerian style is its lack of structure and its emphasis on the development of the individual, which would be at odds with the cultural value of the common good.

Regarding the humanistic-existential approach with its notion of freedom with respect to the issues of control, it is true that Hindus may be limited by their family and it may be difficult to separate individual freedom from the context of the family structure. Many Hindus may value an external locus of control. However, since a value position has been taken that each individual must work out his/her own salvation, existential questions such as "What is man, actual and ideal" and "How can actual man become real," would be fitting.

Jungian approaches that address the "inner stream" would be appropriate because Hindus accept one's innate spirituality and the view that an individual is never an end in himself/herself but always a means toward the development of the real or spiritual self.

Because Hindus come from an elaborate network of social relationships there exists a belief in the importance of harmonious personal relations and a belief that man exists in community. Common welfare is important, and it is for this reason that members of the extended family and kinsmen should be incorporated in the counseling process. Adlerian approaches that focus on the collective spirit fit well with the Hindu value system and stress the welfare of the social group and social interest. Counseling approaches that emphasize individualism and competitive values ignore the importance of socially oriented values in Hindu clients. Adlerian approaches also offer a wide range of cognitive and action-oriented techniques that can help Hindu clients explore their practical problems. These Adlerian approaches, together with other cognitive-behavioral approaches that include rationally definable goals plus the means for the realization of these goals, are fitting. Hinduism accepts that man must of practical necessity live in a world that makes demands and that there is a social obligation to fulfill the demands. Such concrete, tangible approaches are particularly fitting with respect to the Hindu tradition of organizing, classifying and thereby understanding persons in relation to family, society and abstract values.

Hindus have also been conditioned to self-help methods and self-training through the system of yoga, meditation, etc. Counseling approaches could utilize these techniques. Biofeedback techniques also could be used. Emphasis can be placed on inner resources and a heightened self-control of the will. Whatever changes are suggested must fit in with the sociocultural environment.

Hinduism is both mystical and practical at the same time and counseling approaches must address this in treatment approaches. It must be realized, however, that the difference in Hinduism versus Western society is that the ultimate goal is consciousness or awareness, whereas for the West the ultimate goal is achievement. Hinduism is fundamentally concerned with a way of achieving enlightenment and spiritual salvation. A Western approach emphasizes the resolution of personal conflict, whereas a Hindu approach emphasizes transcending conflict and restoring a sense of harmony and community between individuals and their social environments. The world-view of Hinduism offers a new set of assumptions and values.

Counseling approaches also cannot focus solely on the present, as Hinduism embraces both the past and future in its philosophy. Hindus have a strong conviction of continuity. Accommodation of this time perspective would be needed.

Reality therapy could also be used in that the view of rebirth and karma have a moral value, for they teach that what a person receives in life depends on what he/she makes himself/herself to be. Indian literature also has a strong ethical and didactic flavor. Transactional analysis evaluates cultural injunctions and the basis of such conditioned beliefs. Clients can see connections between behavior and what they learned from their family, examining cultural assumptions and baggage.

It must also be realized that in any therapeutic encounter there are clearly defined roles for every Hindu relationship. In every such relationship a hierarchical system of respectful distance is observed between the younger and the older, and between the less powerful and the more powerful. These roles must be respected in the counseling relationship.

CONCLUSION

In sum, the counselor must assess the Indian client's cultural background, taking into account the degree of acculturation and attempting to understand how the client's cultural background may impact on the counseling relationship. The culturally different counselor must recognize the high value that may be placed on family and on education and the sex role socialization that may have taken place. Important religio-philosophical concepts such as karma must be understood if a true understanding of the Indian world-view is desired. Techniques must be chosen that are appropriate to the client's cultural background and the individual differences of the client must be acknowledged so that stereotyping does not take place.

6

Growing up White and Afrikaner

Although not even the architects of apartheid have been able to develop a clear or scientific basis for categorizing the people of South Africa, in terms of the Population Registration Act of 1950 they were divided into rigid "racial" or "ethnic" groups. The very words used to identify each group are contentious because of the oversimplification they imply. Racial categories are essentially social, cultural and political in nature and rest on the shifting sands of biological heterogeneity. In South Africa the divisions are essentially political and perhaps best seen as "color-castes." At the time of the 1985 census, the total population (including the independent homelands) was 33.7 million, of whom 25.0 million (74%) were African; 4.9 million (15%) were white; 2.9 million (8%) were colored; and 0.9 million (3%) were Asian (Wilson & Ramphele, 1989, p. 23).

Cutting across, but also partly reinforcing, these color-castes are the boundaries of language. Along with a host of languages from Africa, Europe and India, the major languages spoken by the majority are the Nguni dialects and the different forms of Sotho. While English is the mother tongue of only one in twelve (8 percent), it is rapidly becoming the common means of communication as a second (or third) language for the majority of South Africans. One in six South Africans speak Afrikaans as a first language, including the coloreds and the white Afrikaners (Wilson & Ramphele, 1989).

This chapter will focus on the white Afrikaners, who have, with formidable purpose, dominated the country since the National party came into power in 1948. Language plays an important role in this group's ethnic identity, although the group has blurred boundaries and there are important political and ideological subgroups. When a category label exists it does not mean that all members of the group use it in the same way (Louw-Potgieter, Kamfer & Boy, 1991).

HISTORICAL BACKGROUND

The core of what eventually became the Afrikaner people were the Dutch and French Huguenots, who fled the tyranny of their European oppressors in search of religious freedom. As the settlers appropriated more land, a series of border wars with the indigenous Xhosa peoples erupted. The Great Trek into the Northern hinterland in the 1830s, similar to the great American migration westward, was caused largely by discontent with the way the border and cattle disputes were handled by the British colonial authorities. In the interior, the land-hungry Voortrekkers clashed with the network of indigenous black tribes who were then in the throes of an internecine war. This resulted in the rise of the Zulu tribe, who became the undisputed lords of the vast region south of the Limpopo river. The climax of the inevitable clash between the white settlers and the mighty Zulu military machine was the battle of Blood River, a seminal incident in the historical consciousness and collective identity formation of the Afrikaner, reminiscent of such famous analogies in American history as the Alamo or Little Big Horn.

On the banks of a stream later known as the Blood River, the Afrikaners, a few hundred strong, drew their ox wagons in a square and secured the openings with thorn bushes. It has become a cliché that "laager formation"—a rigid closing of ranks—is still the Afrikaner's main strategy in dealing with any perceived psychological threat to the group. The Boer victory over vastly superior numbers of Zulu warriors in 1838 later came to be observed as a Sabbath. Generations of Afrikaner children were raised to hold as an article of faith that their ancestors had been led to settle in Africa by divine intervention. As a Christian people, the Afrikaners were compared to the children of Israel and constantly exhorted to remember their past (Hexham, 1981). Sir Lourens van der Post (1990) observed that for the fugitives from Europe the Great Trek was an expression of the desire to find yet a new world in Africa. The real journey Afrikaners now have to make is to turn to their undiscovered world within. This journey will involve self-discovery and the reevaluation of ideological dimensions of the Afrikaner's world-view. Because ideology has played such a major role in shaping the Afrikaner's history and identity, the following section of this chapter attempts to explain how this came about. Later sections will deal with counseling issues related to the Afrikaner's particular world-view.

IDEOLOGY AND SOUTH AFRICA

Foster (1991) takes the view that there are multiple ideological discourses operating in overlapping or cross-cutting ways to effect the three main forms of domination in South Africa: those based on "race," sex and class relations. The main strands constituting these ideological discourses are: (1) racism, (2) Afrikaner nationalism, (3) apartheid, (4) racist capitalism, (5) patriarchy and (6) conspiracy ideology. These are briefly outlined in the following section.

Racism

Racism begins when one derives the (alleged) cultural characteristics of a given group from its (alleged) biological characteristics (Delacampagne, 1990). More to the point, racism is an ideology that refers to a negatively evaluated representation of certain people and acts as a justification for exclusion and/or domination. According to Foster (1991) the dichotomous discourse of "civilization" and "savages" justified the practice of slavery throughout the world. By the early nineteenth century white domination had been firmly entrenched in South Africa through a combination of slavery, restrictions on free blacks, colonial frontier wars and extermination. European "race-science" was woven into the locally entrenched racism during the late nineteenth century. In the course of South African history it has manifested in many changing forms ranging from "baasskap," "trusteeship," and "influx control" to the contemporary ideas of "separate nations," "cultural pluralism," "ethnicity," "minority group protection" and "first and third worlds" (Foster, 1991). In South Africa the concept of ethnic differences was used by the dominant white minority to justify the creation of separate homelands for Africans.

Afrikaner Nationalism

Afrikaner nationalism has evolved over two centuries as a response to the perceived threats first of British rule, and later of indigenous black people. Leonard Thompson (in Coetzee, 1991) wrote: "If anti-imperialism was the warp of early Afrikaner mythology, its woof was the racism that was then endemic in Western culture" (p. 7). Sometimes the anti-imperialist thread was more visible, sometimes the racist thread. A way to strengthen the cultivation of the symbols and fetishes of a national character is by the addition of racism (Balibar, 1990). The latter has indeed supplied Afrikaner nationalism with a theory, a historical backbone and a spiritual core, culminating in the formation of a "civil religion" entwined with the Calvinist paradigm to mold the Afrikaner's emotional identity (De Klerk, 1975; Foster, 1991). Historical mythologies (often factually inaccurate) were infused into the ideology of Afrikaner nationalism to serve the dual functions of inclusion-exclusion: the mobilization of class and fusion of the politically divided Afrikaans-speakers into a cohesive "volk" (nation), and the maintenance of black subordination (Foster, 1991). Ironically, the very same Old Testament biblical themes that were woven into emergent Afrikaner nationalism later came to animate the thinking of the independent African churches, which articulated the sorrows and hopes of the black people under the yoke of Afrikaner oppression (Hexham, 1981).

Apartheid

A number of young Afrikaner intellectuals, including H. F. Verwoerd, the infamous racist South African Prime Minister, did their doctorates in Germany and the Netherlands in the 1930s and returned full of enthusiasm for the goals and methods of the European Right. Geoffrey Cronjé, a sociology professor at the University of Pretoria, formulated the principles of "just race-apartheid," using pseudoscientific rhetoric and notions concerning the God-given sovereignty of the nation. Predictably, racism led to an excess of purism (Balibar, 1990). Cronjé (in Coetzee, 1991) warned that the "racial diversity" of the planet must be protected from "bastardization" and the "mishmash" of races. The colored was held to present the utmost danger for the European race in South Africa. Only total segregation would forestall disaster, because mixed living and mixing in the workplace were the prime causes of miscegenation. The fear of blood mixing was—not coincidentally—mixed with another motive: the issue of employment opportunities. Dr. H. F. Verwoerd delivered a paper at the 1936 National Congress, in which he argued that poor whiteism existed because blacks had taken the jobs of whites. Hence, blacks should be returned to the "homelands."

Racist Capitalism

Apartheid was entrenched because it was functional to particular alliances between state, capital and white trade unionism, the latter galvanized by the threatening competition of a plentiful supply of cheaper and ultraexploitable black labor (Cross & Chisholm, 1990; Foster, 1991; Louw & Kendall, 1986). During the 1950s Prime Minister Verwoerd developed "grand apartheid," setting in motion one of the most ambitious social engineering projects the world has seen. A mere enumeration of the laws promulgated in the period from 1948 to 1976 affecting race relations runs to 507 pages (Institute of Race Relations, 1978). Harsh, repressive measures were increasingly employed to contain black protest and disobedience. The Christian ethic of granting unto others that which one wants oneself and the strategy that blacks were not inferior but merely culturally different were both abused in order to justify the ruthless security machinery and the forced removal of 3.5 million black people to their "own homelands" (Foster, 1991).

Patriarchy

The original formulation of patriarchal ideology was modeled on the family as it existed among rural Afrikaans-speakers before the twentieth century: numerous sons and daughters headed by a patriarch (Coetzee, 1991). This largely idealized image is the model for the Afrikaner guardianship of black "cultural childhood." Bozzoli (cited in Foster, 1991) has argued that there is a "patchwork quilt of patriarchies" in South Africa, varying across class and racial lines. Black women suffer a triple oppression of gender, race and class, while the white women who employ black women as domestic servants depend on them to alleviate some of their own gender burden. Family roles, sanctified by the Dutch Reformed churches, remain traditional: the male is the breadwinner, the female the homemaker with authority vested in the husband. Machismo is socialized into schoolboys through forced participation in the contact sport of rugby. This game is a shrine of Afrikanerdom. It is played and watched with almost religious fervor, and its inherent machismo is firmly entrenched by the time of military conscription of young males after schooling is completed (Leach, 1989). Compensatory machismo in a society where child rearing is almost exclusively "woman's work" is probably also at work (Segall et al., 1990). In Jungian terms, one could speak of the oppression of the feminine by the power aspects of the masculine principle (Saayman, 1990).

Conspiracy Ideology

Christian fundamentalism played a prominent role in the formation of American radical rightism and the political paranoia of the 1960s (Hofstadter, cited in Grenier, 1992). Conspiracy theory is the result of the secularization of religious superstition in which sinister pressure groups are held responsible for all the evils in the world. Like McCarthyism in the United States, the Communist threat has formed the core of South African conspiracy ideology. The African National Congress and the Pan-Africanist Congress were banned in 1960, were increasingly portrayed as part of the "total onslaught" and were seen as instruments in the hands of troublemakers located in the Kremlin. Local critics, church leaders, academics and trade union leaders, stigmatized as "liberals and their running dogs," were despised as dupes of these alien "hidden hands." Thus a complex social reality was simplistically seen as a struggle between "the powers of chaos, Marxism and destruction on the one hand and the powers of order, Christian civilization and the upliftment of people on the other" (P.W. Botha, cited in Foster, 1991, p. 208). In this way, many authoritarian regimes have legitimized death squads, political assassinations and destabilization. When this happens, civil liberties are crushed, and brutality and barbarism replace the rule of law. This has been true for Chile, Colombia, Romania, Uganda and South Africa. When violence and brutality are perpetuated in the name of Christian civilization, difficult moral, and no less difficult psychological, questions are raised. In South Africa, the collective irrationality of politics and history has been especially disconcerting.

A COLLECTIVE MADNESS?

Some historians of apartheid have claimed that it was a rational response to social developments threatening the privilege of white South Africans. Coetzee (1991) asks the inevitable question: "How short-sighted does self-interest have to be before it ceases to be sane, and how much more short-sighted before it begins to be crazy?" (p. 2). Coetzee (1991) maintains that if madness has a place in life, it has a place in history too, and proceeds to analyze the inherent confusions in apartheid discourse. The true force underlying the fear of blood-mixing might indeed be sexual desire and the denial of desire, coupled with fear and greed. Manganyi (1991) recalls Erikson's concept of "pseudospeciation," the process whereby groups ascribe negative qualities in their own identity to subordinate groups in an attempt at psychic self-purification. However, Coetzee (1991) asserts that what is really interesting lies less in apartheid's nature as a passion than in its power to be transmitted and to transmit itself.

THE INTERGENERATIONAL TRANSMISSION OF APARTHEID AND THE LIFE-WORLD OF AFRIKANER CHILDREN

The following sections of this chapter examine the societal structures and instruments that succeeded in spinning a web of "meaning" around the life-world of Afrikaner children. The ideological foundations of Afrikaner dominations were actively created and maintained through various economic and cultural organizations such as the Afrikaner Broederbond, the Dutch Reformed Church, the South African Broadcasting Corporation, newspapers, companies and especially, the system of Christian National Education (Foster, 1991). The input of each of these on the world-view of the Afrikaner youth will be briefly explained.

The Afrikaner Broederbond

The quest for nationality through racism always leads in practice to the self-selection of an elite, because the "superior" race can by definition never coincide with the totality of the national population (Balibar, 1990). The exclusive Afrikaner Broederbond (Brotherhood) was formed in Johannesburg in 1918 by a group of young Afrikaners disillusioned by their role as dispossessed people in their own country. This secret and highly organized clique of "super-Afrikaners" has by sophisticated intrigue harnessed political, social and economic forces in South Africa to its cause: Afrikanerdom's "ultimate destiny of domination in South Africa" (Wilkins & Strydom, 1978, p. 2). All the major political peculiarities that shaped South Africa into the constitutional oddity it was, bore the stamp of the Broederbond. It has numbered most of the country's cabinet ministers among its members. Nobody could become prime minister unless he came from the organization's select ranks. Through its network of 14,000 members and 1,100 cells, it infiltrated its members into every significant leadership position (Leach, 1989). The state-controlled radio and television network was headed by the chairman of the Broederbond for more than a decade. Scores of newspapers and magazines formed an important part of the propaganda machine. Members included college and university lecturers, school teachers and principals, and many Dutch Reformed Church ministers, who were often also chairmen of school boards. The chancellors and rectors of the Afrikaans universities and teacher training colleges and the moderators of the three main Afrikaans churches were ipso facto members. Lately, the Broederbond has transformed itself into an agency of "verligte" (reform) thinking, its more realistic approach ("pragmatic racism") motivated by the realization that survival of the Afrikaner is contingent on the inclusion of blacks in the political process.

The Federation of Afrikaans Cultural Organizations

A shift from "vulgar" to "cultural" racism (Gilroy, 1990) is clearly seen in the cultural focus that marked the inauguration of the apartheid system, and especially in the formation of the Broederbond controlled "Federasie van Afrikaanse Kultuurverenigings" (FAK) in 1929. More than 2,000 cultural organizations were affiliated with or were established by the Federation. It formed organizations for the hundreds of thousands of postal workers, railway workers and policemen. A priority of this unique network was its campaign to capture the youth. The "Voortrekker" movement—reminiscent of the Hitler Youth movement—was formed in opposition to the Boy Scouts and Girl Guides. Primary school children got drawn into the Voortrekkers, who met every week and at weekend camps. The best were picked for survival and leadership camps and conferences. All Afrikaner school children were subjected to periodic weeklong ideological indoctrination courses in "wilderness schools." No Afrikaans child could pass through the school untouched by the pervasive, intense and well-orchestrated process of indoctrination.

The Dutch Reformed Churches

The Dutch Reformed churches are a highly influential force in Afrikaner society. In the heyday of Verwoerdism, that is, ideologically pure apartheid, they played a pivotal role in promoting its moral acceptance among Afrikaners (De Klerk, 1975; Hexham, 1981; Leach, 1989). In consequence, from the 1960s onward, contact with the World Council of Churches was severed, resulting in decades of increasing isolation and retreat into ideology characterized by quasi-theological apologies for apartheid. During the same era, leading church members had close liaisons with right-wing organizations such as the John Birch Society in the United States and neo-Nazi movements in Europe. During the late seventies and early eighties, the political and securocratic exponents of the "total onslaught" philosophy found ready, willing and able allies in Afrikaner church circles.

Christian National Education

The observation that the Holy Roman Empire was neither Holy, nor Roman, nor an Empire is equally applicable to Christian National Education. In fact it was sectarian, sectional and unashamedly committed to indoctrination (Le Roux,

1986). Religion and nationalism merged in an educational theory that prided itself on its devotion to tradition. Modern theories defining education as an enlightening experience capable of loosening traditional bonds and opening the individual to new experiences were rejected (Hexham, 1981). Separate schools with mother tongue as the medium of instruction were justified on religious, psychological-education and national-cultural grounds for the maintenance of Afrikaner identity (Cross & Chisholm, 1990).

All-white schools included in their curricula a paramilitary component, including activities such as "spiritual resilience," emergency services, citizenship, self-defense, shooting and marching activities. The objectives for the guidance programs included "molding the conscience according to the South African hierarchy of values . . . which should inculcate the aspiration of the white population to guard its identity" (Cooper et al., 1990, p. 9). School psychologists and guidance counselors were specially trained at the white Afrikaans colleges and universities to "spiritually arm" the youth against the onslaught of ideas and ideologies that might undermine the "volk" (Botha et al., 1975). Technology, the women's liberation movement, working mothers, pop music, pornography, modern art, drugs, alcohol, materialistic values, homosexuality and Darwinian theory were equally condemned.

Textbooks

The teaching of history as a school subject played a pivotal role in socializing each successive generation into the ideology of apartheid. Indeed, racism, like Marxism, depends on a historiosophy (philosophy of history): it thrives on an interpretation of history as a "secret," hidden and then revealed to men about their own nature and destiny (Balibar, 1990). South African history was interpreted and represented to result in the construction of the "Afrikanervolk" and its romantic national mythology.

A number of studies (Foster, 1986) have shown that school coverage of South African history textbooks was largely devoted to the history of white groups at the expense of blacks. Blacks were presented as obstacles to the achievement of white objectives, and the legal and moral authority of the whites as not questioned. The country "rightfully" belonged to the white Afrikaner. This kind of tunnel vision education meant that information was depicted in terms of the symbolic system of whites and was always supportive of the status quo. Although empirical demonstration of such influence is not available, there seems little doubt that school textbooks are likely to influence the process of political socialization and the development of racist ideology (Foster, 1986). Coetzee's analysis of apartheid discourse reveals how subtly, insidiously and pervasively the ideological discourse permeated every aspect of the Afrikaner child's life-world. In the following discussion of counseling implications of the Afrikaner child's world-view, the focus will be on these particular ideologically related issues. More general counseling issues need not be exploited here, because in other respects the Afrikaner child's counseling problems do not differ substantially from those associated with mainstream Euro-American culture, nor are suitable counseling approaches different from those that would be useful for white, middle-class youth in other societies.

AFRIKANER WORLD-VIEW AND COUNSELING ISSUES

Sir Lourens van der Post (1990) said that apartheid did not set out with the conscious idea of being malignant. Rather, it did set out with quite wrong assumptions, which were bound to have appalling consequences. For decades the all-pervading mood of South Africa's social nexus was characterized by fear, depression, rage and doubt (Saayman, 1990). As patriarchal politics insidiously inserted itself into every aspect of life, the very words "South Africa" provoked passions that reverberated with universal outrage at such racial domination. South Africa came to cast the shadow of the world. This "shadow" was cast on the geographically and socially divided life-world of Afrikaner children. The symptoms of racial indoctrination are discussed in the final section of this chapter. To see these in perspective, however, the deep divisiveness and inequality of the South African society must be borne in mind.

Perhaps the most striking feature of the South African society is its inequality. There is a gulf between "grinding poverty and massive wealth" (Wilson & Ramphele, 1989, p. 17). In 1987, South Africa's Gini coefficient (which measures inequality) was the highest of any of the fifty-seven countries in the world for which data were available. In 1980, the proportion of Africans, who comprise the dominant population, living in poverty was estimated to be nearly two-thirds (60.5%). In contrast, whites, who are a very small minority, earned about two-thirds of all income.

There is a stark contrast between the beauty of most suburbs, where privileged white South Africans live, and the townships inhabited by blacks. White children play in parks geared to safety while township children play in busy, hazard-ridden streets. Even in the "dorps" (towns) of the "platteland" (rural areas) the environment is very different in black and white areas. In Hanover, for example, the white section of town is a pretty place with furrows of water running down the sides of the tarred streets and beautiful, huge trees offering shade against the scorching sun. The other part of town, for blacks only, "makes one sweat before entering" (Wilson & Ramphele, 1989, p. 133). The importance of the spatial attributes of social conduct should not be underestimated and Le Roux (1986) emphasizes the effect of geographical and social apartheid in accounting for the success of the National party's political indoctrination of Afrikaner youth. South Africa thus represents a world of contrast, resulting in the Afrikaner world-view characteristics discussed below, for example, ethnocentrism, anxiety and fearfulness, stereotyping and alienation, ignorance and rationalization, intellectual incarceration, a warped world of values and distorted racial-cultural identity development. Each of these is briefly elaborated upon in the following sections.

EARLY ETHNOCENTRISM

If the Broederbond, the churches and the National party were not entirely successful in imbuing the children with the puritan work ethic and strict sexual morality they envisaged, they were more successful in their ethnic mobilization of the Afrikaner. "The philosophy of separate development was swallowed as readily as good koeksisters" [a traditional confection] (Le Roux, 1986, p. 199). Studies concerning political socialization help to explain this success. Also, what was taught in school was echoed in the home. The family may indeed be a more important agent of political socialization than the school or the peer group (Le Roux, 1986). The point is that young Afrikaners grew up in an atmosphere of pervasive and unquestioned racism.

Moodie's 1980 study (reported in Foster, 1986) found an increasing awareness in white children between the ages of six and thirteen of Afrikaans/English group identity. At age six more than half drew pictures of their family in response to the request to "draw the people of your country." By age thirteen all of them had progressed to a sociocentric stance and drew pictures depicting racial groups or public scenes, but, significantly, nearly half of the white, English-descendant adolescents drew only black figures, whereas none of the white Afrikaner children did so. Ethnocentrism was rife and led to an earlier and closer identification with national symbols such as the flag and the national anthem. There was, as well, a largely uncritical attitude toward the government in Afrikaner children compared with English-speaking youths who traced their heritage to the United Kingdom.

ANXIETY AND FEARFULNESS

Gibson (1990) emphasizes the impact of the pervasive societal violence on white children: the states of emergency, the security legislation, the bomb threats, the increasing militarization of all aspects of society, and the subtle and diffuse fear of "the black danger." It must be borne in mind that children are subject to the power of their imaginations. They are able to construct elaborate fears and fantasies based on limited information, picking up the subtle signs of fear and concern in the adults around them. A case study of "Daniel," an eight-year-old white boy, poignantly underlines the complexity of questions regarding individual versus collective guilt when it comes to children who, although materially advantaged by it, cannot be held responsible for the injustice of the society into which they were born (Gibson, 1990).

STEREOTYPING AND ALIENATION

Melamed (Louw & Foster, 1991) showed that basic features of racial differentiation and stereotypes were established by the age of six years. Unlike young black children who tend to show outgroup preference and identification, white children show strong ingroup preference. Barling, as well as Moodie (Foster,

1986), found that ethnocentrism increased with age for children aged seven to twelve. Orpen and Pors (Segall et al., 1990) investigated social distance in white, middle-class Afrikaans-speaking teenagers. The findings showed race to be more important than belief congruence in determining social distance. The basic psychological determinant of social distance is perceived similarity, but when racial discrimination is officially sanctioned, this masks individual psychological tendencies. However, many psychological factors (authoritarianism, dogmatism, field dependence) may influence intergroup relations and behavior, attitudes toward outgroups are subject to institutionalized norms and other forms of social control (Segall et al., 1990).

Hodge (1990) maintains that oppression in all its forms is sustained by an ancient moral concept: the dualism of good and evil. Afrikaner children were taught to justify oppression of blacks as part of the struggle between the forces of good and evil. The victims were seen as bad or as motivated by evil. By extension, the treatment of their victims was not viewed as oppression at all, but as justified—a victory of good over evil. The notion that all human beings are of equal worth was deliberately stamped out in educational theory and practice by placing it somewhere on the continuum humanism-liberalism-egalitarianism, which in turn was associated with Marxism-atheism-satanism.

IGNORANCE AND RATIONALIZATION

A frequent defense of the status quo was that Africans in South Africa were better off than people in many other Third World countries. Even children "knew" that in those countries in which blacks were getting independence, chaos immediately set in and, besides, local blacks could exercise all their rights in their "own" homelands (Le Roux, 1986). Such rationalizations existed by the grace of ignorance. Very few white children had any knowledge of how blacks were progressively excluded from political and economic spheres and the repressive measures used to achieve this. Even today, few whites believe that African pupils are educationally worse off than their counterparts elsewhere (Pillay, 1990).

Roland Barthes (1990) penetratingly describes how easily simplified, "common sense" notions concerning the black world can be confirmed by the popular press. Collective representations have been kept stagnant and children kept impotent to imagine the black other. The stresses involved in supporting the "laager mentality" were sometimes overwhelming. When cracks appeared, that is, personal inadequacies or problems coalesced with a general feeling of insecurity, Afrikaners directed their frustrations against those closest to them and caused scores of deaths through family murders (Leach, 1989).

INTELLECTUAL INCARCERATION

The effect on Afrikaners of their own xenophobia, as well as their ostracism by the civilized world, led to a time-warp effect in their world-view. Afrikaners' lives became politically and mentally incestuous, a rigid adherence to received norms. The intrusion of the modern world into an existence that has remained largely undisturbed for three centuries was not easily tolerated or absorbed (Leach, 1989). Indeed, the humanities at Afrikaner universities tend to reflect nineteenth-century European world-views. Appiah (1990) is correct when he says that racism is often associated with a kind of "cognitive incapacity"—an inability to give up beliefs that play a part in justifying the special advantages whites have gained from their positions in the social order. Racists exhibit a systematically distorted rationality. However intelligent or otherwise well informed, they fail to treat evidence against the theoretical propositions of racism dispassionately, resulting in a distorted value hierarchy.

WARPED WORLD OF VALUES

In 1986 Joe Lelyveld noted that an Afrikaner could go surprisingly far in those days without reading himself/herself out of the establishment. The Afrikaner could theorize on issues such as land reform or income distribution and could draw constitutional models that looked like chandeliers or DNA molecules. Likewise, he/she could even theorize about the likelihood of negotiating one day with the (at that time still) banned black political groups. What the Afrikaner could not do was appeal to values such as justice and equality. Only then did he/she become a renegade. It was "politically quite immoral" to appeal to justice and the "fairness factor," according to an editorial in an influential Afrikaner newspaper, without the smallest trace of irony, because that could only mean "surrender to black power" (Lelyveld, 1986, p. 73). Justice might demand that the door be opened to black power, the newspaper was saying, but black power would be inherently evil. Therefore, justice was immoral. In this way, generations of Afrikaans grew up with a warped hierarchy of values built into their social-cultural identity.

DISTORTED/ARRESTED RACIAL-CULTURAL IDENTITY DEVELOPMENT

Sue and Sue (1990) describe the progressive stages of identity formation displayed by whites in a racist society. Their white identity development model would seem to be equally applicable to South African whites. Its basic assumptions certainly hold true in that racism is an integral part of South African society and that all whites are socialized into this society and inherit its biases. The phases of white identity development are similar to the phases through which a black person may move: conformity, dissonance, resistance and immersion, introspection and integrative awareness. The implications of Sue and Sue's model in the South African context are as follows:

1. Much of the material in the previous sections of this chapter merely affirm that many, if not most, Afrikaners have been deliberately entrapped in the conformity stage.

Apartheid education has created ethnocentricity and a bloated sense of identity as well as an incapacity to conceive of different social relations. It has bestowed on the white psyche the expectation of rights and privileges that are considered sacrosanct (Nkomo, 1990). Typically, there is minimal accurate knowledge of other groups, but a great deal of adherence to stereotypes. The stage is also marked by the sometimes baffling, contradictory, but compartmentalized attitudes, beliefs and behaviors described under previous headings.

2. The white person moves into the dissonance stage when forced to deal with these inconsistencies and/or encounters information or experiences at odds with previous denials.

This leads to a radical self-examination of values. Adolescents and young adults are the ones most likely to recognize their racism and the part they themselves play in oppression. Leach's (1989) book on the Afrikaners indudes a number of compelling autobiographical accounts of the events and experiences that have triggered this stage—especially the violence of 1976, the banning of black organizations a year later and the detention of leading black activists, such as Steve Biko who died in police custody. In fact, Leach suggests that the Afrikaner's widespread political confusion during the eighties signified a collective dissonance stage.

3. Resistance and immersion is characterized by strong anger toward family and friends, institutions and societal values, which are seen as having sold the person a false bill of goods. Racial self-hatred may be experienced.

The "white liberal syndrome" may develop, resulting in the paternalistic protector role or in overidentification with the oppressed group. Leach (1989) describes the moral pilgrimages of a number of "wayward sons of Afrikanerdom," who deserted the "volk" and fled into exile to join the ranks of the African National Congress (ANC). Many were sentenced to imprisonment for terrorist activities.

4. The introspective stage is marked by a need for greater individual autonomy and a realization that feelings of guilt and anger are dysfunctional. The person no longer denies that he or she is white, but seeks a more balanced stance.
5. When the integrative awareness stage is attained, a sense of self-fulfillment with regard to racial-cultural identity is experienced.

A self-affirming, but nonracist white identity emerges, with pride in those aspects of white culture that are nonexploitative. The person can now acknowledge responsibility for perpetuating racism, but is no longer immobilized by guilt or prompted into rash acts by anger. There is increased knowledge of sociopolitical influences and racial relations, increased appreciation for cultural diversity and increased commitment toward eradication of racism. Counseling implications and the broader educational challenges posed by this ideal are elaborated in the final chapters of this volume, while the special counseling issues of racist values in children and youth are only briefly touched on in the final section of this chapter.

COUNSELING IMPLICATIONS

Delacampagne (1990) rightly warns that if it wants to be effective, the ideological struggle against racism should not be inspired either by a desire for mortification or by a crazed need for self-punishment. It should not have the perverse effect of leading us to deny the real diversity, biological and cultural, existing within the human species, nor of making us sink into a total cultural relativism. Cultural relativism would imply that the normative imperatives, in the name of which we combat racism, are themselves arbitrary. In the words of Manganyi (1991):

> Racism is about difference. A series of attributes have been used in the past to proclaim racial difference, and apartheid as we have come to live it and support or resist it, as so many have done—is a local variant of a human weakness on a tragic and grand scale. This is the universal story of treachery and innocence. (P. 1)

In regard to the children who are the inheritors of privilege and distorted cultural identity, Victor Hugo's words (quoted by Pauw, 1991) come to mind: "If a man sins because of darkness, the guilty one is not he who sins, but he who causes the darkness" (p. 98). Appiah (1990) contends that the racists in a racist culture resist rational control or reasoning. Such people should not be treated as morally responsible for their acts reflecting racial prejudice. In Appiah's (1990) words:

> It is a bad thing that such people exist; they are in a certain sense, bad people. But it is not clear to me that they are responsible for the fact that they are bad. Racial prejudice, like prejudice generally, may threaten an agent's autonomy, making it appropriate to treat or train rather than to reason with them. (P. 9)

From a system perspective, all Afrikaner children and youth have been the products of a racist society. This aspect of Afrikaner identity will more than likely emerge in counseling sessions.

In reeducating South Africans, the notion of "racial formation" (Omi & Winant cited in Outlaw, 1990) should replace the idea of "race" as an "essence," that is, as something fixed, concrete and objective, or alternatively, as a malignant illusion, which in the ideal social order should be eliminated. The notion allows an appreciation of the historical and socially constructive aspects of "race" within the context of a theory of social evolution where learning is the central feature. Social learning regarding "race" might help us to move beyond racism, without reductionism, to a pluralist democracy. We must acknowledge the "other side" of "race": the lived experience of those within racial groups, especially those blacks for whom black nationalism is fundamental. We have to appreciate the integrity of those who see themselves through the prism of "race." We must not err yet again in thinking that "race thinking" can or must be completely eliminated on the way to an emancipated society (Outlaw, 1990).

CONCLUSION

South Africans must strive toward democracy in a multiethnic, multicultural society where, for better or for worse, cultural diversity and group thinking will remain decisive features of social and political life. In facilitating growth and development, counselors who work with Afrikaner clients must understand a world-view that has included early ethnocentrism, anxiety and fearfulness, stereotyping and alienation, ignorance and rationalization, intellectual incarceration, a warped world of values and a distorted racial-cultural identity development.

7

The Shaping of Colored Identity

In his introduction to *Pedagogy of Domination,* Nkomo (1990) explains why in that particular volume the term "black" is used to refer to all of the oppressed groups in South Africa, namely, Africans, coloreds and Asians (e.g., Indians). The reason is that the political and social consciousness of the oppressed groups has produced a common self-definition that expresses their desire to unify in the struggle to abolish apartheid. Indeed, the very existence of a separate and identifiable colored population is questionable. The Colored People's Convention in 1961 declared that "a Colored person is one who is discriminated against in a particular sort of way" (Lemon, 1987). Many colored intellectuals refer to themselves as "so-called coloreds." Goldin (1987) argues that racial divisions in South Africa represent the outcome of an intense battle being waged at all levels of society between competing ideologies. These divisions are in a state of flux; the movement reflects the changing balance of forces in the struggle to mobilize racial identity.

Nevertheless, and however distasteful this may be, disaggregation of the generic term *black* (into African or black, colored and Indian) is necessary to facilitate the description of the full and differential impact of apartheid on the various groups. Some of the effects of apartheid have been unique to this group due to their particular, ambiguous situation vis-à-vis both the white and the black groups. Care should be exercised in dealing with the opposition between the abstract concept of what the world *should* be like and the reality of the world as it is (Saayman, 1990). There is a danger of obscuring realities in the name of ideals.

BACKGROUND

The colored people of South Africa represent more or less 8 percent of the total population (Wilson & Ramphele, 1989). At the time of the 1985 census, they numbered about 3 million out of a total population of approximately 34 million. The Malays, who are of Eastern origin, form a special subgroup constituting about 18 percent of the population. They are Moslems much influenced by the beliefs and values of their faith (Gillis, in Van Zyl, 1990). Nearly 90 percent of the colored population live in the Cape Province, where rapid urbanization has contributed to their concentration in metropolitan areas, although many live and work on white-owned farms. In spite of the fact that in many districts they actually outnumber the dominant white population group, they remain socioeconomically and politically repressed and marginalized. There are small communities in the Orange Free State and Natal, while Johannesburg has its own colored settlement area called Eldorado Park located on the doorstep of Soweto, similar to the colored area outside Pretoria, called Eersterust. Eersterust is located between the white suburbs of the capital city and Mamelodi, a sprawling black township housing the African work force who commute to Pretoria's business and industrial hub every day. The geographical location of this colored settlement, situated between the white and black areas, is an apt metaphor for the psychological and social location of the colored group, hovering on the social borderline between the white and black groups.

SITUATED ON THE RACIAL BORDERLINE

The marginal position occupied by the colored group must be understood as part and parcel of the Afrikaners' attempts to reconstitute society in order to guarantee their supremacy. Successive governments have tried to develop a client group, who although not assimilated into the dominant class, owe it their allegiance. The development of the colored group was part of such a process. But the forging of colored identity cannot simply be attributed to the state and to the ruling class: The colored population also defined itself. From the outset, colored identity was an area of conflict. The term *colored* was rejected by many of the people so defined, while others imputed a different meaning to the term. It became the focus of a passionate debate. This has increased in intensity over time and the term has become overloaded with connotations which invariably invite confusion and criticism (Goldin, 1987).

It cannot be stressed enough that many, if not most, people in South Africa reject the racial categorizations imposed on them by apartheid legislation. The term *mixed race* reproduces in another form many of the racial prejudices inherent in the now discarded National party view that coloreds were largely the result of miscegenation between the European settler population and the indigenous inhabitants of the Cape colony. Although such intermixing has undoubtedly contributed substantially to the population defined today as colored, it was a nonsense attempt to distinguish the colored people in this manner. "Mixed race" implies the prior existence of "pure" race-groups and gives credence to apartheid notions of racial purity. No race exists that is not mixed, least of all the supposedly pure English (Anglo-Saxon) race or the "white" Afrikaners with their exotic potpourri ancestry (Goldin, 1987). The coloreds in South Africa constitute an artificially created "ethnic group"—a creation of the racially obsessed white dominant group (Coetzee, 1991; Outlaw, 1990). Nevertheless, ironically and as a bitter testimony to the brutal efficiency of apartheid, a significant degree of social identification within the colored group has developed. It is particularly apparent at the ghetto level. As a result of the loss of the middle class through emigration, a social dichotomy has developed—the intellectual elite, ideologically committed to a nonracial society—and the gravely disadvantaged, acutely aware and jealous of their "differences" from their African compatriots.

EFFECTS OF STATUTORY APARTHEID

Since 1948, when the Afrikaner came to power, the colored people have been forced to live in separate colored areas and to use only their own, vastly inadequate, public amenities. They were barred from participation in the social and cultural life of mainstream white society and deprived of meaningful participation in the governance of their country of birth. This state of affairs was created and maintained through a series of repressive laws. It is impossible to understand the life-world of the colored people of South Africa without understanding how some of these laws shaped their lives.

According to the Population Registration Act, a person is a colored if he/she is not a white or a Bantu (African). In its turn, the category colored is subdivided into the Cape colored group; the Malay group; the Griquas; Chinese; Indians; other Asians; and other coloreds. The accumulation of negative definitions caused the coloreds to feel that they were merely a residual group—coloreds are what is left over when no other category fits.

Classification of a person was determined by "derivation." In the case of a child born to a mother and a father of different ethnic groups, the child was classified as belonging to the natural father's ethnic group. Thus a child might be raised by a colored mother and live in a colored community, but be classified as a "Bantu" if the father was African. These laws caused intense humiliation and sometimes tragedy (Leach, 1989). Some members of a family might have been classified as white and others as colored on the basis of spurious scientific and biological analysis. There were numerous borderline cases: Individuals accepted by their community as white were suddenly labeled as of mixed blood.

Perhaps the worst trauma was caused by the laws prohibiting "mixed marriages" and "immorality" (sexual intercourse between the races). These laws—repealed only in 1991—raise serious moral and religious questions. The harm done by them to the relationships between white, colored and black people will take many years to be healed. The implication behind these laws was felt to be that a colored person is so inferior to a white that sexual relations or a love relationship culminating in marriage were immoral and criminal (Leach, 1989; Lemon, 1987).

The laws pertaining to group areas, land tenure and separate amenities caused no less damage. The philosophy of separate group areas was, according to its architects, meant to prevent "friction" between the different groups, who were often allocated dormitory areas separated by buffer zones like railway lines, hills, valleys or rivers. To achieve the desired degree of separateness, large communities were uprooted from neighborhoods or townships they had occupied for generations and relocated.

Up to 1976, more than 75,000 colored people were thus forcibly removed, causing untold hardship and harm to community and family life, as well as to human dignity (Platzky & Walker, 1985; Theron & Du Toit, 1977). Often the relocation areas were barren plains or windswept valleys hidden behind a hill. Out of sight of the city, the colored workers continued to earn a living, which entailed long hours and costly journeys by public transport to get to work. Families were split up, bereft of their familiar support networks and neighbors. They were dumped in rows of identical tiny houses, where simple amenities like food stores, tarred streets, pavement, water, sewage facilities and electricity were often inadequate or absent. Community and recreation centers, post offices, parks, libraries, churches, public telephones and police stations often took years to be built.

The rezoning of District Six in Cape Town, and the forced removal of close to 35,000 people who had lived there for generations, to make way for white-owned industry and business, is the most notorious example of this kind of social engineering (McCormick, 1986). Lemon (1987) describes how numerous business enterprises were destroyed in the process. Ironically, private enterprise has largely declined to purchase the dispossessed land and so become associated with "tainted land." District Six has therefore remained an empty shell—a symbol of the hurt and distress caused by forced removals. In the words of Franklin Sonn, a respected educator and leader: "The Group Areas Act killed my people—economically and morally" (in Leach, 1989, p. 227). A colored person interviewed by the Theron Commission expressed the feeling of dispossession and alienation in these words (translated from Theron & Du Toit, 1977, p. 14): "It is bitter to be an outcast in the country of your birth." Another interviewee said: "We have no country of our own—we have only no man's land." The question to be addressed in the following section is whether this dispossessed and alienated group possesses a unique cultural heritage and identity. Particular attention will be paid to language, community life, education and family structure as dimensions of the "colored culture."

COLORED CULTURE

The Theron Commission (Theron & Du Toit, 1977) found that the only real differences between white and colored groups were ethnic and socioeconomic and that culturally the two groups were virtually indistinguishable. The ethnic contrast between the white and colored groups has been ruthlessly maintained by a white group fanatically proud of its racial purity. This sector was pathologically afraid of "intermixing," and created legislation that prevented sexual relations and cohabitation or marriage across the color bar. The socioeconomic differences have been deliberately maintained by way of repressive legislation. Culturally, the colored people are far more similar to the Afrikaner than the African or Indian groups, although Leach (1989) observes that their wit, humor and exuberance under extremely adverse circumstances distinguish them from the more dour, Calvinist Afrikaner. Perhaps the clearest way to explain the subtle cultural differences and similarities between the two groups is to examine the images and values associated with language.

LANGUAGE

Describing the use of language in District Six (where colored people have lived since 1818), McCormick (1986) stresses the complex information conveyed by the choice between Afrikaans and English. This choice provides information about the speaker's actual or desired position on a number of parameters such as regional background, social class and political or religious affiliation. The adults interviewed by McCormick were very aware that the Afrikaans that they use is different from "pure" or standard Afrikaans. They referred to their own dialect as "broken" or "kitchen" Afrikaans. It is a dialect of Afrikaans characterized by a high degree of code-mixing: English words, phrases and sentences are liberally interspersed with nonstandard Afrikaans forms. The English loan-words are often altered to fit Afrikaans patterns, while pronunciation may be modified, thus producing a highly distinctive, colorful and expressive blend.

An ambiguous sense of cultural identity is reflected in the mixed feelings of colored people in regard to their use of Afrikaans. They feel that outside of their own speech community it is bound to evoke stereotypes of laziness, lack of education and poverty. At the same time, the Afrikaans vernacular is the language of intimacy and friendship within the community. Although many people are able to speak standard English as well as standard Afrikaans, in informal situations they slip into the comfortable vernacular. The use of either of the standard dialects would be seen as a deliberate signal of distance.

The use of standard Afrikaans has mixed connotations. A colored person heard to speak it might be taken for an unsophisticated country person (since Afrikaans is used by most rural colored people), or else seen to be progovernment (a "sell-out"). Standard Afrikaans is often called "the language of the oppressor" because of the strong association between Afrikaner nationalism and apartheid. Significantly and sadly, only a very small minority of the colored persons interviewed by McCormick (1986) who classified themselves as Afrikaans-speaking, was able to express undivided, unambiguous love of their mother tongue. Recently, the dialect has been relabeled "Cape Afrikaans" and ingroup speakers have changed the evaluation of Afrikaans from "the language of the oppressor" to "the language of struggle against oppression" (Louw-Potgieter, 1991).

The English language is a marker of upward social mobility. English is associated with city life, good education, good work opportunities, middle-class lifestyle and access to the world outside South Africa. Many Afrikaans-speaking coloreds, disgusted by apartheid, distanced themselves from their original ethnolinguistic group by anglicizing (Louw-Potgieter, 1991). The confident use of English is also seen as a challenge to whites who may stereotype coloreds as uneducated, especially if the white person addressed is not proficient in English. In the words of a colored Afrikaans-speaker interviewed by McCormick (1986): "If I speak to a Colored, I speak Afrikaans. And if I come across a native [African] and he can speak Afrikaans I speak to him in Afrikaans. If I come across a white I like to speak English because most of them don't like it" (p. 295).

Regarding the linguistic choices provided for the children in the colored community she studied, McCormick (1986) found that English was the preferred language for bringing up children, even in homes where the adults usually spoke Afrikaans and were not very competent in English. A typical explanation given was the following (translated from Afrikaans): "Look, I don't want my children to be like me. I want them to be better than me. Right?" (p. 296).

Parents feel that a good command of English will give their children access to better educational and job opportunities and enable them to assert themselves in a discriminatory society. Consequently, many parents prefer their offspring to go to English medium schools. Often these children are disadvantaged, due to the difficulties of coping with the demands of school in an unfamiliar language. Many have to acquire not only a second language but also a second dialect upon entering school. They are expected to develop competence in the standard dialects of both official languages. Simultaneously, they have to remember to keep the two languages separate in formal school discourse, while the vernacular that they use at home and in the neighborhood draws on both languages. McCormick (1986) found that although some children find it difficult to follow instructions in English, they will not ask questions for fear of showing that their English is not adequate. At home, their parents may drill them to maintain the appearance of being English-speaking in order to be eligible for the "English stream" in school. Not surprisingly, there are scholastic difficulties. Worse problems result if correction of deviance from the standard dialect is not handled with great tact. It can give the children a very negative image of themselves and their homes, or even render them self-protectively mute. Thus the loyalties and divisions that exist on a sociopolitical level create academic hurdles.

COMMUNITY LIFE

Social problems within the colored community are intimately linked to economic and political circumstances that have been largely beyond the control of individuals and groups. Over generations such adverse circumstances can erode the will to plan for the future to such an extent that both physical and psychological health are undermined (Cilliers, 1971; Theron & Du Toit, 1977; Wilson & Ramphele, 1989). Gastroenteritis, a fair reflection of a community's socioeconomic status, especially regarding its children, is the most common cause of death in the colored community (176 per 100,000). The corresponding figure for whites is 4 per 100,000 (Wilson & Ramphele, 1989). Colored children manifested significantly higher incidences of psychiatric disorder than white children (Van Zyl, 1990). Families and communities have been living below the breadline for generations. For these people, planning for the future becomes impossible. The struggle for day-to-day subsistence consumes all the energy they have. Children do not aspire to a higher educational level than their parents, most of whom did not make it through primary school.

The very high incidence of crime in the colored communities is reflected in the relative representation of coloreds in the prison population compared with other groups. In the year 1982–1983, the number of prisoners was 3,527 per 100,000 population in the case of coloreds and 2,475 for Africans, but only 476 for Indians and 392 for whites (Lemon, 1987). Drunkenness was by far the most frequent cause of convictions, followed by assault and various forms of theft. Such crimes are indicative of a low level of feelings of human worth and dignity, which are clearly related to the marginal position of coloreds in the wider society. The disruption of family and community life wrought by forced removals and resettlements was one of the primary causes of criminal behavior. Very often, newly settled communities had to wait years for a police station in the neighborhood. Because there were few if any public telephones, police could not be summoned to report a crime. Consequently, gangs often ruled neighborhoods made up of narrow, ill-lit streets and crowded tenements.

Alcohol and drugs played a prominent role in the crime statistics. Marijuana was often consumed along with alcohol, becoming a highly volatile combination that easily leads to violent behavior (Theron & Du Toit, 1977). According to Lemon (1987) the "tot system," whereby colored farm laborers have been traditionally paid in wine, still survives. The fact that licensed premises were not easily accessible to colored farm workers also encouraged a buying pattern of weekly acquisitioning with heavy consumption over weekends, when for most there is no alternative recreation. Both alcoholism and the smoking of "dagga" (marijuana) reflect the search for immediate gratification in the face of underlying frustrations. Retreat is also found in religion, with many coloreds attracted to emotional worship in small churches with a strong emphasis on individual salvation. These evangelical churches appeal to many coloreds in much the same way that they once attracted poverty-stricken white American farmers in the Appalachian Mountains (Lemon, 1987).

Children who grow up under circumstances in which they are exposed to violence and crime, even deliberately socialized to participate in it, face a bleak future. In school they are mostly too old for their standard, chastised by teachers and taunted by peers because of their dirty and ragged appearance. Inevitably they play truant, form gangs and soon drop out of school, often joining the numbers of "strollers" or street children who roam the cities in search of some form of shelter and food. A closer look at the colored education system throws additional light on the high early drop-out rate.

EDUCATION

Scholastic progress and education have been impeded by factors such as overcrowded classrooms and a shortage of qualified teachers. The teacher-to-pupil ratio is approximately 1:29 and only 6 of every 100 students graduate from high school (Fitzgerald, 1980). Approximately one-third of the teachers have not graduated from high school and only 4 percent have a university degree (Livingstone, 1989). In some magisterial districts, schools up to Standard 4 (Sixth Grade) are available to most children, whereas in others, even in the 1980s, there was virtually no provision of schools. In the Hanover district of the Karoo, for example, the only colored school in a district where 30 percent of the population lived in rural areas was in the town (Wilson & Ramphele, 1989). There were no colored farm schools and only one for Africans. In the magisterial district of Calitzdorp there are twelve farm schools and one large primary school in the town. However, there are no high schools for colored pupils in the entire district. Those who do reach high school are forced to go to the neighboring town of Oudtshoorn. This means a drastic increase in the family's monthly outlay for items such as boarding fees and transport costs for home visits. It is little wonder that there is a significant drop in the number of those with more than eight years of schooling. In one survey, it was found that the proportion of those who were functionally illiterate (with no more than six years of schooling) were 45 percent in Bergsig, the colored township of Calitzdorp, and 80 percent on the farms (Wilson & Ramphele, 1989). Along with disrupted community life and inadequate educational provision, family breakdown is another factor contributing negatively to the colored child's life-world.

FAMILY STRUCTURE

Most colored households consist of a father, mother, one or more unmarried children and a number of other persons, such as married children and their offspring or other members of the extended family. However, the problem of overcrowded living conditions is exacerbated by the housing shortage, the lack of institutional care for persons in need of care and the aged, the high incidence of extramarital pregnancies and the need for parents to leave younger children in the care of somebody when both go out to work (Theron & Du Toit, 1977; Wilson & Ramphele, 1989). A large percentage of households are headed by a mother as single parent, the high incidence of extramarital and teenage pregnancies being a contributory factor. The Theron Commission found that 33 percent of all colored children were born out of wedlock, while more than 80 percent of infants were born to mothers below the age of twenty (Theron & Du Toit, 1977). The commission concluded that it was nearly impossible to maintain "normal" standards regarding marriage, sexual morality and child rearing in the face of the prevailing poverty, overcrowded living conditions and alcohol abuse. In 1990, Van Zyl still found a high incidence of severe problem drinking, mostly among fathers with a lifestyle involving weekend drinking combined with discord and assault. Sadly, drinking patterns seem to remain remarkably stable, and the link between psychiatric disorder in children and severe drinking by fathers remains significant. It is perhaps not surprising that an oppressed group afflicted by the debilitating effects of divided cultural loyalty, disrupted community and family structures and poor education and poverty, is also subject to the negative effects of stereotyping by the dominant group responsible for much of their misery.

STEREOTYPING

The Theron Commission (Theron & Du Toit, 1977) found that whites tend to indulge in massive denial, rationalization and projection when they are confronted with the "colored problem." Western (in Lemon, 1987) summarized the elements in the white image of coloreds that have led to feelings of impotence and racial inferiority because they may have been internalized by colored people or may have caused intense resentment:

1. White "possession" of coloreds is exemplified in master-servant relationships and the names given to coloreds by slave owners that survive today as family names.
2. The juxtaposition of coloreds' classification as mixed race and prohibition of mixed marriages, coupled with the Afrikaner's quasi-religious horror of miscegenation, implied that coloreds are impure, immoral creations (Coetzee, 1991; Hexham, 1981; De Klerk, 1975).
3. The musical image is related to troupe-style entertainment, together with the image of coloreds as happy jesters, both of which are deeply resented by politically aware coloreds.
4. The stereotype of coloreds as being sexually *proliferate* relates partly to the tradition of whites seeking illicit pleasures in colored areas of Cape Town (District Six, Mowbray).
5. Perhaps the cruellest stereotype relates to the oppressor's image of the oppressed as being poor, unambitious and ignorant, and therefore undeserving of the privileges enjoyed by the ingroup, forgetting the very oppressive measures implemented by the Afrikaner to keep the coloreds poor, unambitious and ignorant (see Hodge, 1990).

The negative impact of internalized stereotypes and the accompanying feelings of inferiority and resentment have probably contributed in no small way to ambiguous ethnicity and problematic identity formation in coloreds. The next section elaborates on these phenomena and counseling issues related to the colored worldview.

AMBIGUOUS ETHNICITY AND IDENTITY FORMATION

As stated previously, there is a racial and political colored awareness, mainly because "persons of color" have been considered as different by whites almost since the first settlers arrived in 1652 (Lemon, 1987). Four decades of apartheid have magnified whatever collective awareness already existed. On any criteria other than those of descent and physical characteristics of race, coloreds belong to the white population from whom they are partly descended and whose language and culture they share.

There is a definite advantage in being fair-skinned and straight- or light-haired, particularly if one can "pass as white" (Lemon, 1987). If coloreds wanted the good things in life, they had to "try for white." The only other option was to emigrate to a country where skin color did not play the pervasive and pernicious role it played in the land of their birth. From the early sixties to the end of the seventies, many tens of thousands of middle-class coloreds chose the emigration route to self-fulfillment. Tragically, this resulted in the typical ghetto syndrome, which is also familiar in the United States. Those who could have upgraded the community life and served as role models of success to the next generation leave the country. At the same time, there was the "internal emigration" of those with sufficient intelligence, training and initiative (contemporaneously blessed with a sufficiently light complexion) to the ranks of the whites.

In 1976, when the Erika Theron Report was submitted to Parliament, it was stated that only 50 to 70 percent of the colored population indicated that they were proud to call themselves colored. However, the Theron Commission already warned that the positive sense of identity was on the wane, especially among the higher socioeconomic strata and the younger generation. It was also noted that even amongst those coloreds who evidenced positive identification with their group, this should not be taken to mean that they accepted the negative status accorded to coloreds in the society characterized by statutory discrimination and racism. The reasons given by those who did not accept their ethnic identity included the following: "My skin is not colored"; "It makes me think of hardships"; "One feels branded"; "It refers to second-class citizens"; "It gives the impression that we are mixed," and, "We did not ask for it" (Theron & Du Toit, 1977, p. 95). It is easy to understand why Franklin Sonn (Leach, 1989) describes his people as "possibly the angriest community among the South African population" (p. 227).

Using a social distance scale, Rakoff (in Foster, 1986) tested over 500 colored adolescents between the ages of twelve and fourteen during the late 1940s. Results showed that they felt most tolerant of their own group, followed by the Malay group. However, the third most favored group was English-speaking whites, while they evidenced little if any solidarity with fellow oppressed blacks. A high degree of intolerance was shown toward Indian, African and Chinese, all rated as less acceptable than Afrikaans-speaking whites. In contrast, the attitudinal color bar was strongly evidenced by a white adolescent sample who rated all white groups as more acceptable than any other group.

According to the Theron Report, some colored communities in areas where they were forced to share "non-white" areas with black and Indian inhabitants, insisted on their own, exclusively colored "group areas," following the example of the white population in their fear of being "swamped" by the other groups (Theron & Du Toit, 1977). This desire signified the wish of a significant percentage to identify with the white group.

In the Western Cape, the National party pursued a deliberate policy of preference of coloreds regarding employment and residential rights in order to mobilize colored racial identity (Goldin, 1987). The preference policy was closely associated with attempts to deflect opposition based on the alliance of colored and African workers. The enforcement of influx controls over Africans extended the relative advantage of an assertion of colored identity. Attempts to undermine the alliance of African and colored people were not entirely successful. There was increasing resistance of coloreds to a separate colored political identity during the sixties and early seventies. For many coloreds, increasingly disillusioned by the failure of white and colored politicians to advance their position, the only way forward was for their joint organization with black South Africans. The attempts of the state to undermine nonracial organizations have been resisted by liberation movements and trade unions. These organizations are committed to the promotion of a democratic and nonracial society; in striving for this goal they have been engaged in a long and bitter struggle against racial identity.

COLORED WORLD-VIEW AND COUNSELING ISSUES

Evidence exists that the development of the colored personality has been severely handicapped by the sting of apartheid. Lambley (1980) found that of all three groups studied (Afrikaans, English and colored), the colored person's personality structure was the most fragile. They knew and understood the reality imposed by the Afrikaner because they had more contact with it. According to Lambley, psychometric findings on the Minnesota Multiphasic Personality Inventory (MMPI) and Rorschach tests indicated that the profiles of colored males came close to peaking on the schizophrenic scale and colored females scored significantly higher on the scales measuring depression, schizophrenia and hypomania. The colored male and female profiles were very similar to each other, indicating a similar level of defensive functioning and style of personality. Lambley (1980) attributes this to the belief that personality development was not shaped according to sex stereotype, but to apartheid. He felt that the pattern of response was the manifestation of extreme stress and not the fact that colored subjects were psychotic or even borderline, but that they were deeply stressed. As a result of prolonged exposure, they had to develop ways of coping that in any other culture would be regarded as psychotic or borderline. Tremendous fears and anxieties were to be found in this reality and they had accurate perceptions of the dangers facing them. To attend to these perceptions led to survival, but at the price of having to maintain a chronically disturbed personality. In other studies of coloreds Lambley (1980) performed using projective techniques, he found them to register high on oppression, victimization and helplessness.

According to Sue and Sue (1990), minority groups who have consistently been victims of discrimination and oppression in a culture that is full of racism have good reason to be suspicious and mistrustful of white society. Under these circumstances "cultural paranoia" may be healthy and adaptive rather than dysfunctional and pathological. Indeed, the absence of a "paranorm" among minorities may be more indicative of pathology than its presence. The absence of a paranorm may indicate either poor reality testing (denial of oppression-racism) and/or naivete in understanding the operation of racism. In this context, the concept of marginalized personality development has been raised.

A MARGINAL PERSONALITY?

The term *marginal man* (person) was first used to describe a person who finds himself/herself living on the margins of two cultures and not fully accommodated to either. It was once thought that the marginal position in which colored people find themselves would lead to the development of a "marginal personality" characterized by feelings of insecurity, self-pity and exaggerated sensitivity. However, research during the 1950s done under the supervision of Gordon Allport did not support the hypothesis of a "marginal personality" amongst the colored population (Louw & Foster, 1991). Research findings have emphasized the complexity of factors in marginality. Because it became doubtful whether it was useful to speak of a marginal personality, research based on marginality theory petered out after the mid-1960s.

There is, of course, nothing inherently pathological about bicultural membership, but marginal individuals are thought to be characterized by an external locus of control and an internal locus of responsibility (Sue & Sue, 1990). (Locus of control refers to people's beliefs regarding the cause of success or failure, e.g., contingent on their own actions, or determined by chance or luck. Locus of responsibility refers to the degree of responsibility or blame placed on the individual as opposed to blaming the system.) Marginalized persons are most likely to accept the dominant culture's definition of self-responsibility and to deny the existence of racism. They have probably internalized the dominant group's stereotypes regarding themselves. They may evidence racial self-hatred, unconditionally accept white social and cultural standards, and perceive physical features of white men and women as an exemplification of beauty. They are powerless to control their sense of self-worth because approval must come from an external source. As a result, they are high in person-focus and external control (Sue & Sue, 1990).

The marginal position and status thus may affect the colored individual's total orientation toward self and others. These detrimental effects are not the results of internal dynamics, but of the social system. The inequities and injustices of apartheid have caused many coloreds to manifest an external locus of control coupled with a external locus of responsibility. Such a stance is high on system-blame. The person feels that there is very little he/she can do in the face of such external obstacles as prejudice and discrimination. This response might be a manifestation of having "given up" or an attempt to "placate" those in power. In its extreme form, oppression may result in a form of "learned helplessness" associated with passivity and apathy in the face of underemployment, unemployment, poor quality of education and poor housing. These persons may fail to learn that there are events that can be controlled (cognitive disruption), and may show anxiety and depression (emotional disturbance).

Growing up in a world caught between a privileged white group and a less privileged black group may be assumed to be detrimental to normal development of the intra- and interpersonal relationships in children. A child was reported by the Theron Commission of inquiry into the position of the colored population in South Africa (Theron & Du Toit, 1977) to have summed it up in these words (translated from Afrikaans): "My head spins since apartheid came in. What does it mean?" After it had been explained to him, he responded: "The white folks don't like us, so we have to live apart" (p. 9). Research is needed to clarify the interrelationships among psychological and social factors producing stress, alienation from the larger society, marginality and other intrapsychic conflicts.

STAGES OF RACIAL-CULTURAL IDENTITY DEVELOPMENT

The task for coloreds, despite these many barriers, is to develop pride in their racial and cultural identity. Identity development represents a process of self-actualization. Sue and Sue (1990, pp. 95–112) have proposed a five-stage Racial/Cultural Identity Development model (R/CID) that may be used as a conceptual framework to aid counselors in understanding the colored client's attitudes and behaviors. The model defines five stages of development that oppressed people experience as they struggle to understand themselves in terms of their own culture, the dominant culture and the oppressive relationship between the two cultures: conformity, dissonance, resistance and immersion, introspection and integrative awareness. At each level of identity, corresponding beliefs and attitudes are an integral part of the minority person's identity and are manifest in how he/she views (1) the self, (2) others of the same minority, (3) others of another minority and (4) majority individuals.

A colored person in the conformity stage may manifest unequivocal preference for the dominant white group, deprecate the colored group and show discriminatory attitudes toward blacks and other minorities. Many colored clients may be expected to be in the dissonant stage of identity development and will manifest conflicting attitudes and beliefs regarding self and others of the various groups. Likewise, many coloreds are in the resistance and immersion stage, characterized by guilt, shame and anger because of having been a "sellout" in the past. An introspective phase is ideally followed by the final, integrative awareness stage, where minority persons have developed an inner sense of security and now can own and appreciate unique aspects of their culture, as well as those in other cultures. At the integrative awareness stage, the minority person has a strong commitment and desire to eliminate all forms of oppression. Surprisingly, many colored persons in South Africa have already reached this stage.

The Black Consciousness (BC) movement had a profound effect on racial and cultural identity development in many coloreds. Its philosophy gave the coloreds a new sense of dignity. One colored man said in this connection: "Today I can see that I also am a flower in God's garden" (Leach, 1989, p. 229). The BC movement was an important catharsis for the colored people. In Franklin Sonn's words: "To us, Black Consciousness was a real and emotional experience. We discovered ourselves. It gave us a sense of pride after the years of alienation. We could at last tell ourselves that we were free of . . . the Afrikaners and all that hardship and rejection, and callous, unfeeling racism" (Leach, 1989, p. 229).

Full acceptance of the colored child by the community could depend on the child's acceptance of an African identity and involvement in the African struggle for liberation. In a study conducted by Lasovsky (in Foster, 1986), colored women in the Western Cape were divided into two groups, high and low awareness of black consciousness. Self-esteem measures were obtained from mothers and their children, whose ages ranged from six to nine years. The "high aware" group of mothers scored higher on the self-esteem measure than the "low aware" group. The same trend was found for the children, although the results were not highly significant.

Having found their own identity, many coloreds returned to the search for a common, nonracial South Africanism as reflected in the Freedom Charter drawn up in 1955. To achieve a nonracist identity, they first had to go through black consciousness to discover themselves. Despite the hurt suffered under apartheid, the coloreds would dearly love to be the vehicle to guide the Afrikaner towards a new future, to help him fulfill a creative role as a true South African. The coloreds' role might well be to free the Afrikaners: "We have a mission to take them into Ubuntu [African humanism]. We have a mission to shake them loose from their racism and their inward-looking nationalism" (Sonn, quoted by Leach, 1989, p. 229).

COUNSELING IMPLICATIONS

Sue and Sue (1990) warn that the historical and current experiences of racism and oppression are likely to cause some healthy suspicion in the victim's attitude to a culturally different counselor. Insofar as the educational guidance movement has had an impact on colored schools, it is not unfair to say that in many instances it has been used as an oppressive instrument by those in power to maintain the status quo. Within an apartheid education system, counseling services may indeed be an unjust and cruel exercise of power to subjugate or mistreat people by way of overt and covert forms of prejudice and discrimination. The colored client's world-view may well boil down to one central question when confronted by a white counselor: "What makes you . . . any different from all the others out there who have oppressed and discriminated against me?" (Sue & Sue, 1990, p. 6).

Bearing in mind the remarks on the "paranorm" above, the traditional counseling and therapy process in which the client is expected to talk about the most intimate aspects of his or her life, may cause difficulties. Colored clients may be initially reluctant to self-disclose, thus placing them in a position whereby they may be judged to be mentally unhealthy or "paranoid." Communication may be further hampered by the complex interrelationship between language and status, and power and social class factors discussed earlier in this chapter. A "culturally encapsulated" counselor (Sue & Sue, 1990) may, because of blindness to his/her own sociopolitical baggage, ignore the fact that the use of "objective" psychological tests may place repressed minorities at a disadvantage. The colored child may be especially vulnerable to unfair comparison with privileged white children of the same age.

Conversely, if the client is characterized by marginality and self-hate (external locus of control and internal locus of responsibility), a white counselor might be perceived as more competent and preferred to counselors of the client's own group. For this client, focusing on feelings may be very threatening, since it may reveal the presence of self-hate and the realization that he/she cannot escape from his/her own racial and cultural heritage. A culturally encapsulated white counselor who does not understand the sociopolitical dynamics of the client's concerns may unwittingly perpetuate or intensify the conflict. Therapeutic processes and outcomes are often the function of the identity development stage of both counselor and client (Sue & Sue, 1990).

In the context of the South African history of racial discrimination and oppression against coloreds, the counselor should at all times guard against the possibility of "blaming the victim." This may happen if, adhering to white, middle-class notions of individual responsibility originating from an ideological milieu of individualism, the counselor were to ascribe failure to the client's lack of ability, interest, maturity or some other inherent weakness. This would be especially detrimental if the client has developed an expectation of helplessness. An effective counselor would realize the basis for this adaptation and would teach such clients new coping strategies, help them to experience success, and validate who and what they represent. The colored child (and his/her family) has probably been subjected to high stress factors in society and placed in a one-down position by virtue of racism. The lifestyle of colored communities can only be portrayed as inferior, underdeveloped or deficient in the absence of a broader systems analysis showing that the economic, social and psychological conditions of minorities are related to their oppressed status.

CONCLUSION

According to Franklin Sonn (Leach, 1989) the coloreds and the Afrikaners were on the same social and economic level in the 1920s and the 1930s. Both were impoverished. In reviving their own fortunes, the Afrikaners simply pushed the coloreds out of the system. This caused a great deal of anger. Nevertheless, the colored people still yearn to be reacquainted with their Afrikaner compatriots, but not at any price. Politically, many may identify with the black struggle, but deep down the desire is strong to forge a common nationalism and a cultural reassociation between white and colored Afrikaners. The two groups have much in common: their language, their religion and, often, their looks. Yet those coloreds who neither identify with whites nor with blacks are probably the majority. They want only to be identified as South Africans. They are opposed to any form of ethnocentrism or racial prejudice. They abhor statutory discrimination on the grounds of ethnicity. In this, they join the mainstream of modern Western value systems.

Part III

Psychological Trauma in Childhood and Adolescence

The material in this section (chapters 8 and 9) describes the disempowerment of children and youth in South African society as a result of apartheid. The consequences of poverty and the effects of violence are the contexts within which the majority of children must cope, and a generation of maladjusted children may be the result. In South Africa, social and economic conditions have had a major impact on mental health. The effects of poverty, injustice and racism have not only failed to promote good mental health but have been specifically detrimental to its attainment. Racism has undercut the roots of healthy mental life by depriving children and youth of a sense of self-esteem, freedom for personal growth and identification with a community of equals. Accordingly, many South African children and youth have either witnessed the violence of civil war or have been subjected to the violence of the apartheid system. There may be psychic numbing, a sense of meaninglessness and little hope for the future. Because of these factors, a sociopolitical approach has been adopted and is based on the premise that much of the aberrant behavior in children and youth is rooted in the existing pathology of social conditions rather than in the pathology of the individual. The authors recommended that mental health workers become involved in education, housing, employment and other issues that can affect intervention strategies and programs. A community-based approach should be adopted and the following chapters provide a base for understanding environmental influences and for program design and service delivery. That which has yet to be attained is a healing culture that will promote the growth of all South Africa's citizens.

8

Child Abuse in South Africa

There are a number of features peculiar to South African society that color the forms of child abuse in perhaps unique ways. These South African peculiarities are mostly related to the degree to which the government has resorted to direct legal intervention to organize the most personal details of people's lives (Burman, 1986). For example, the Population Registration Act, No. 30 of 1950, and Proclamation 123 of 1967, introduced no less than nine categories into which people had to be classified. The main divisions were "white," "black" (African) and "colored," the latter in its turn subdivided into "Asians" (subdivided into Chinese and Indians), and "other coloreds." Until 1985, sexual relations and marriage between whites and members of other groups were forbidden, punishable by prison sentences. The implications of social engineering of this kind must be a major concern of mental health workers. The legacy for the future is twofold: the material deprivation suffered by the underprivileged groups, and the stereotyped and hostile attitudes with which children, totally isolated in segregated communities, have been imbued (Burman, 1986).

Nevertheless, what is peculiar to South African variations of child abuse may shed new light on the more common manifestations, particularly by highlighting the universal fact that abuse is always embedded in a series of interlinked contexts ranging from the family and the community to larger social, economical and political contexts. The South African experience is a reminder that the mechanisms of power in a society and the phenomena of repression or exclusion have their instruments and their logic at the effective level of the immediate environment, of the most basic units of society, that is, classrooms, families, parents and children (Burman, 1986). The South African experience has also demonstrated how these phenomena even spill over the boundaries of national borders, as neighboring countries (Angola, Mozambique, Namibia, Botswana and Zimbabwe), which form part of the same geopolitical and economic complex, impinge on each other's histories. This is especially true in the case of a society characterized by pervasive and intense degrees of structural violence—which have plagued South Africa.

STRUCTURAL VIOLENCE

According to John Galtung, who first coined the term, structural violence is "present when human beings are being influenced so that their actual somatic and mental realizations are below their potential realizations" (Degenaar, 1990, p. 11). The violence may be built into the structures that do not give the citizens equal power and equal life chances. A just society is a developed society, and social justice may be defined as equal treatment of persons. When this equality is withheld from citizens, the term *structural violence* can be applied to the state of affairs. Paternalistic and selective development are also cited as examples of structural violence. Selective development can also be a mechanism for structural violence by arbitrarily depriving certain areas of possible development. Following this line of argument, one may say that any institution that systematically robs certain people of rightful options generally available to others, does violence to those people.

When rulers enforce oppressive and discriminatory laws without the consent of the ruled, structural violence may be characterized by the worst kind of political injustices. In terms of the definition of structural violence, South African society has been regarded internationally as the worst example of a structurally violent society. It has probably been the only society on earth that legally enforced discrimination, with all the connotations of inequality and injustice associated with this term. Degenaar (1990) quotes Allan Boesak, who speaks of an unending spiral of violence inherent in the apartheid system:

> South Africa has been a violent society with violent laws defended by violence. The implication is that structural violence invites physical violence. This view is held by some revolutionaries as a justification for the use of physical violence in liberation movements. The spiral is completed when police and military forces respond with yet more effective physical violence.

Structural violence manifests itself in the uneven distribution of power and resources. It manifests itself when resources and powers are unequally shared and are mainly the property of a restricted number who use them not for the good of all, but for their own profit and for the domination of the less favored. In such a context, even peaceful laws that help maintain this order may be seen as instruments of violence (Degenaar, 1990). Perhaps the worst manifestation of the structural violence inherent in South African society is the pervasive abuse of its children and youth.

A CHILD-ABUSING SOCIETY

Seen in its historical perspective, the assumption of power by the National party in 1948 marked not so much a turning point in South African history as the intensification of processes that had been going on for 300 years. Nevertheless, some of the special policies pursued by the National party government have created a society that has been in its very structure a person-destroying and child-abusing society. The policy of apartheid not only fostered conditions conducive to child abuse and neglect, but was and is in itself abusive. The state is the ultimate guardian of the young, and therefore has a responsibility to ensure both their physical and emotional well-being. When the state enacts laws keeping large sections of the population destitute, poorly educated and in disrupted families, it not only fails to promote the well-being of the children in its guardianship, but fosters conditions, which in themselves, are conducive to child abuse and neglect (Straker, Moosa & Sanctuaries Counselling Team, 1990, hereafter Straker et al., 1990).

It is true that children are often socially invisible and do not appear in the pages of most history books (Burman, 1986). Along with women, children form one of the "muted groups" in a society when it is seen at a distance. However, because they reinvent and transmit the values of society, they affect profoundly the patterns of behavior and the attitudes of that society. A society that abuses its children is abusing its own future. Apartheid's structural assault on children has been waged in a variety of ways (Wilson & Ramphele, 1989). These include:

1. The creation of "reserves," "homelands" and "independent self-governing states" whereby millions of people were impoverished by excluding them from the industrial economy protected by the apartheid borders.
2. The prevention of black urbanization rested on the philosophy that blacks should only be allowed into the towns as temporary workers and was achieved by three techniques: pass laws, the limitation on housing construction, and the destruction of "squatter communities" which were formed near the white cities. Each one of these mechanisms had profound and devastating effects on the quality of family life and human dignity, inevitably spilling over into the lives of those most vulnerable to poverty and social disorganization: women, the elderly and, especially, children.
3. The crushing of organizations whereby people excluded from the right to vote might have exercised their potential power on the South African political economy. This has resulted in the banning and breaking of countless political movements, trade unions and student organizations. Adults—many of them parents—cannot be arrested, jailed, beaten up, banned, exiled, or marginalized and radicalized without creating a cascade of spill-over effects on their children. The erosion of authority structures in the family where the father is humiliated and brutalized by the police in his own home under the eyes of his children has also negatively impacted on children.

4. It is often overlooked that the effects of apartheid did not stop at the borders of South Africa. Through various tactics, the South African government over several years has carried out a policy of destabilization in the neighboring countries of Angola and Mozambique. Untold misery was caused for families and children by warfare, terrorism, sabotage and destruction of health, education and community structures. The carnage has been indiscriminate, with infants and children not exempted. Apart from the deaths caused by bullets and bombs—also witnessed by children—thousands more died from famine, malnutrition and disease indirectly caused by the military destabilization.

RACIAL DISCRIMINATION

Racial segregation, an important child-abusing mechanism in South Africa, has a long and infamous history (Straker et al., 1990). A pass system restricting the freedom of movement of blacks was first introduced by the British in 1809. The official policy of apartheid, euphemistically called "separate development," was introduced by the National party when it assumed power in 1948. The government then instituted a system of political and social control based on racial discrimination and aimed at maintaining the political, economic and cultural dominance of the white minority. Under this system, laws were enacted restricting the areas in which blacks could live, creating a situation of unequal educational opportunities and placing a ceiling on occupational skills and economic opportunity for blacks. Thus, blacks have been kept in a position in which they are mostly impoverished, poorly educated and frequently unemployed.

Nobel Peace Prize laureate Bishop Desmond Tutu (Burman & Reynolds, 1986) succinctly described what it means to be born into an apartheid society:

> Depending on your pigmentation, you are placed high or low on the social pyramid; and where you are or, rather, where your parents are, determines so many things for you. It will decide, with a rigidity unknown even in the strictest Calvinistic predestination, where you are born and where you can live. It will determine what sort of health care is available to you; indeed, it will determine your chances of survival or whether you will become part of the dismal infant mortality statistic. . . . It will determine whether you can ever hope to be treated as a human person of infinite worth because you have been created in the image of God (pp. xv–xvi).

Dowdall (1990) stresses the less obvious—the debilitating effect of the undermining of self-concepts and self-confidence by the hundreds of devaluations black people had to suffer—and still have to suffer—in a system in which they were constructed as inferior and less capable and held in impotent roles. The destructive force of the white man's construction of blackness is poignantly described by Fanon (1990), but it is difficult to estimate the shame and self-contempt that may be generated in children by witnessing their parents' humiliation and submission. It seems that feelings of anxiety and/or inferiority in relation to ethnic identity may be formed before children are four years old (Group for the Advancement of Psychiatry, 1987).

POLITICAL SUPPRESSION

The apartheid laws impacted children and adolescents more indirectly than those passed more recently under the State of Emergency. These latter laws allowed large-scale detentions without trial, legitimized the presence of the army and riot police in large numbers in townships and generally contributed to young people being directly exposed to high levels of violence. Straker and her associates (1990) posit that whereas it may well have been accused of child neglect through its earlier laws, the later laws lay the state open to the accusation of active child abuse. As in political struggles elsewhere, children have often borne the brunt of state repression. Early protests by children against the inferior black education system were met with violent repression. This set up a vicious cycle of further protests, boycotts and stonings of police vehicles, which was followed by police using tear gas, rubber bullets, whips, shootings and detentions on a huge scale. Several hundred schoolchildren have been shot and killed in these protests. The New York–based Lawyer's Committee for Human Rights have labeled the situation a "war against children" (Dowdall, 1990). South African children have participated in street battles and have been involved in violent acts toward those members of their own communities regarded as "sellouts" or collaborators with the state (Dawes & Tredoux, 1990).

Obviously, all these young people experienced various levels of stress before, during and after these events. However, the effects of political suppression are not only directly experienced, but also indirectly. Gama (1990) describes the effects of children's incomprehension of—and adults' inability to explain—the absence of family members who were in detention or in hiding, police searching people's homes, soldiers patrolling the streets and schools being teargassed. Children reacted with symptoms of anxiety, fearfulness, tension, withdrawal, sadness and depression. Some children became hypersensitive and/or hyperactive and displayed conduct disorders. Common symptoms were school refusal, school phobia, aggressive behavior, running away from home and defiance toward parents, adults or authority in general. An increased rate of teenage suicide was reported.

Klaasen (1990) further refers to the following kinds of state-inflicted and government-endorsed violence: jails for children; the separation of families through detentions; the harassment of whole societies; and the presence of the army in residential areas. All of these had a psychological effect on children, yet there were also severe physical forms of violence inflicted on children: they were shot, murdered, maimed and raped by police, soldiers and such agents as "witdoeke." One may add to the list of perpetrators politically inspired youngsters as well as politically camouflaged gangsters and thugs. The same author (Klaasen, 1990) describes how 500 people were treated for gunshot wounds at the Empilisweni Sacla Clinic in Crossroads in the nine-month period from February to November 1985. Of these, 41 were younger than fifteen years, and 118 were between the ages of fifteen and twenty.

Malepa (1990) describes vividly how the South African Defence Force's presense in the urban townships—patrolling the streets in casspirs or hippos (armed military vehicles)—caused anxiety and fear in preschool children. The sight of the police and the army were identified with violence and not protection. Black children tend to relate to whites not as human beings, but as enemies. Even very young children display violent behavior in their drawings and games. Thato, a three-and-a-half-year-old boy, could give step-by-step directions for making a petrol bomb. Especially distressing to educators like Malepa was the destruction of family life and the apparently pervasive loss of respect for life. Klaasen (1990) and Clowes (1990) confirmed the fear that children were becoming familiarized to violence without understanding the issues in question. Many children have found it difficult to handle situations of violence in which they have been involved. It has emerged that some of the children who have been drawn into acts of necklacing (i.e., placing a tire that has been doused with gasoline around a victim's neck and setting it alight) have had nightmares, while others have been admitted into mental institutions and still others have taken to drugs. Especially in this context, the sale of toys like machine guns, tanks and army kits is an additional source of concern.

DETENTION

In a massive wave of political detentions, more than 55,000 people were imprisoned under states of emergency and security legislation in the four years leading up to March 1988 (Gibson, 1990). During the second State of Emergency, in July 1985, 8,000 people were detained, of whom about 2,000 were under the age of sixteen (Dowdall, 1990). During the third State of Emergency, some 10,000 youths under the age of eighteen years were detained (Dowdall, 1990; Gama, 1990). Under the pressure of an international outcry, the detentions were subsequently limited and, in 1988, the number fell below 500 children. However, many young people remained in hiding or "on the run" for years. At the height of the widespread and sometimes indiscriminate detentions, not only activists, but also politically unconnected people were arrested in large numbers. Commonly, these were youths between the ages of fourteen and nineteen years, who were picked up at home, in school or from the streets. They were frequently assaulted during the arrest and sometimes further abused at the police station. Reports of physical torture, including electric shocks, were frequent, as were threats of hanging or burning. Children were held in overcrowded cells, sometimes in the company of common criminals. Many were held in solitary confinement for long periods. The anxiety and uncertainty experienced during these processes were pervasive and exacerbating factors. Youngsters were not told why they were being held or for how long. Parents were seldom, if ever, notified and spent distressed weeks searching hospitals, mortuaries, police stations and prisons for their missing children. The psychological effects on the families have been, in many instances, devastating—notably manifested in disillusionment, fear, hatred, feelings of powerlessness, separation and emotional loss, guilt and clinical depression (Robertson, 1990).

The common symptoms observed by Dowdall (1990) and his associates in young people released from detention had many of the features of posttraumatic stress disorder, with underlying anxiety and depression. The most common and long-lasting problem was disturbance of concentration, often associated with lapses in memory that sometimes emerged as "blanks" in conversation. The youngsters had difficulties in "putting someone's words together." Not surprisingly, this led to scholastic difficulties. Sleep disturbances were common, often accompanied by vivid nightmares. Also recorded were flashbacks, startle reactions and extreme emotional responses to cues connected with detention, for example loud knocking, or a harsh tone of voice. Emotional numbness and a sense of emptiness were reported by youths who had been seriously abused, as were physical aches and pains and frequent headaches or stomachaches. Also common were interpersonal problems such as irritability, erratic and inappropriate emotional responses and a sense of alienation in relationships. With older teenage males, sexual difficulties such as impotence occurred.

CONTINUOUS TRAUMATIC STRESS DISORDER

The diversity and multiplicity of trauma to which many black youths have been directly exposed resemble those described by researchers working with children during World War II, and more recently, by those working with children in Northern Ireland and Israel (Straker et al., 1990). However, some South African psychologists have questioned whether "posttraumatic stress disorder" accurately describes the condition of South African victims of oppression and violence. For example, many ex-detainees are not in a limited stress situation that ends with release (Dowdall, 1990). Many youths were exposed to multiple trauma including witnessing death, being arrested, being beaten, being in exile and being separated from family and friends (Straker et al., 1990). Thus, a pattern of ongoing harassment emerged, in which the police burst in on people at any time, and questioned, threatened or redetained them. The victims suffered the additional stress of ostracism by the local community who wanted to avoid "trouble" or were actively hostile to the ex-detainees. Teenagers were excluded from school by the school principals. In some cases, the victimization was continued by black vigilante groups who threatened, abducted, injured or even killed ex-detainees or members of their families. The detention survivor could never afford to let defenses drop and had to live a deeply unsettled life, often "on the run" for long periods of time. It is not surprising that such youths often manifested chronic and generalized suspiciousness, deep feelings of hatred and anger and severe depression. Hence, it seems more apt to speak of continuous traumatic stress disorder rather than posttraumatic stress disorder.

One striking difference between youths who may be suffering from continuous stress disorder and individuals studied under posttraumatic stress conditions is the degree to which the former freely express anger, hostility and revenge fantasies, while the expression of fear is inhibited. According to Straker and her counseling team, this finding parallels that of Punamaki, who worked with Palestinian children on the occupied West Bank (Straker et al., 1990). This phenomenon may be explained in terms of social pressure, which disallows the expression of fear and encourages overt aggression when people see themselves as engaged in ongoing conflict. The mobilization of aggression in a war situation has a survival value. This does not mean that fear is absent—individuals in the group studied by Straker and associates (1990) betrayed their anxiety by sleep disturbance, nervousness, irritability and tics. The victims' perception of the cause of their problems was a complicating factor during counseling, for example, the belief that they were bewitched by their enemy's witch doctor or that they were haunted by the ghost of a murdered loved one. Upon analysis, these beliefs often had a masking function—either masking unacceptable wishes or survivor guilt. Also, the location of causality outside of the self, as in bewitchment, may serve to alleviate feelings of blame and guilt.

FORCED REMOVALS

During the twenty-three years from 1960 to 1983, an estimated number of 3.5 million people have been forcibly removed from one place to another in order to fulfill the apartheid planners' schemes for racially segregated living areas in the cities, towns and villages of South Africa (Wilson & Ramphele, 1989). Old people and children were among the hardest hit by the shock and hardships of dislocation. A less obvious effect of the Group Areas removals—was the destruction of the ties that bound communities together. The fabric interlinking generations was often destroyed. The Second Carnegie Commission (Wilson & Ramphele, 1989) reported the following first-hand account:

> It was like a man with a stick breaking spider webs in a forest. The spider may survive the fall, but he can't survive without his web. . . . Before, there was always something that kept the community ticking over and operating correctly . . . there was the extended family, the granny and grandpa were at home, doing the household chores and looking after the kids. Now, the family is taken out of this environment where everything is safe and known. It is put in a matchbox in a strange place. All social norms have suddenly been abolished. Before, the children who got up to mischief in the streets were reprimanded by neighbors. Now there's nobody and they join gangs because that's the only way to find friends. (P. 143)

Dawes and Tredoux (1990) documented the emotional sequelae for children of the Crossroads incident, arguably South Africa's most brutal forced removal. One mother reported that her children sleep under their beds with their clothes on. If someone knocks loudly on the door, they climb out of the window and run away. Significantly, many children were highly ambivalent toward the police, not being able to decide whether they were law enforcers and protectors or enemies of the struggle.

EDUCATIONAL DEPRIVATION

South Africa has the doubtful distinction of being one of the countries in the world where children have invaded the arena and the history books usually reserved for adults. The Children's Crusade of 1212 and the Cambodian children of the Khmer Rouge come to mind as similar examples (Burman, 1986). In South Africa, starting with the boycotts in 1976 and escalating to the breaking point in the mideighties, schoolchildren have been at the epicenter of a political storm lasting for nearly two decades and raging throughout the country (Wilson & Ramphele, 1989). With astonishing courage, the children put "liberation before education." Stones were no match for whips and bullets. Many children were arrested and held in solitary confinement. Some were tortured and released traumatized. Many paid with their lives.

The price of the children's revolt also had to be paid in lost educational opportunities. Many children lost two, three or more years of schooling. Amidst the turmoil, some never went to school at all. A whole generation lost years of education that cannot be recovered. Those who grew up without schooling have suffered perhaps irreversible loss.

DISINTEGRATION OF FAMILY LIFE

Until recently, laws governing where black people could reside often prohibited families from living together. A breadwinner may have been authorized to reside near the workplace, but the rest of the family may not have been (Straker et al., 1990). Although the infamous Group Areas Act prohibiting blacks from living in the choice areas reserved for white people has been repealed, systematic economic disadvantage perpetuates separate living areas. Blacks are still forced to live far from their places of work, entailing long hours on buses and trains and contributing to a poor quality of life. Many workers arise between 3:00 and 4:00 A.M. in order to reach their place of employment by seven or eight o'clock in the morning. They only return home long after their children have gone to bed. Overcrowded and depressing townships, low work status, and dangerous and crime-ridden environments create tensions in family living that often lead to a high alcoholism rate and family violence (Dowdall, 1990). However, for those black families confined to the impoverished "homelands," the outlook is even bleaker for family life. To survive, the father is commonly forced to become a migrant laborer, leaving his family for six months or a year at a time. This system has had a devastating, fragmenting effect on nuclear and extended families, the traditional sites of childcare. It has been estimated that two out of every five African men working in South Africa are migrant laborers (Dowdall, 1990).

Women and children suffer the heaviest burdens of uncertainty and fear due to the risks of family breakdown under the migratory labor system. A woman in Qua-Qua told the Second Carnegie Commission (Wilson & Ramphele, 1989): "When the father is gone he forgets about the children" (p. 158). A Gazankulu wife added: "Men often do not care for their families. When they come back at Christmas or Good Friday, they do not bring anything to their family" (p. 158). Many children are born of young mothers whose husbands are away working in the cities as migrants. The instability of family life, for which the migrant labor system must bear much of the blame, is a major factor in infant mortality and childhood malnutrition.

Even if the husband is monogamous and does not have a second wife or family in town, the costs of living separately are higher. Few migrant workers can live apart from their families year after year without building up a second circle of friends and relationships, which in turn involves spending some money on them (Wilson & Ramphele, 1989). This money is deducted from what little can be sent home to the wife and children in the reserve or homeland.

Divorcees and deserted wives often find themselves destitute because of a society structured in such a way that women are financially overdependent on their menfolk. For example, the right to a house in an urban area could, until recently, be forfeited by a woman who became divorced from her husband. In addition, divorcees trying to secure maintenance of their children from former husbands or, worse still, common law husbands, have to contend with such difficulties that few of them ever succeed.

Because most of the better-paying jobs are in the hands of men, the degree of poverty is far higher among female-headed households than in homes headed by a man. In some areas, more than half of the households are headed by females (Wilson & Ramphele, 1989). The special twist given to poverty by the racist and sexist laws and practices of the state, exacerbated by the traditional sexism of the tribal cultures, make the position of black mothers, unsupported by menfolk, grindingly hard to endure. All of this impacts on the children, who are the real hostages taken in the war.

INADEQUATE CHILD-MINDING AND PRESCHOOL FACILITIES

Another problem is the absence, particularly in the urban areas, of adequate child-minding and preschool facilities. Economic necessity has forced large numbers of mothers to seek employment. In a climate of high unemployment, many mothers are forced to return to work very soon after the birth of their babies, often before the child is two months old. In one study referred to by Straker and her associates (1990), it was found that 50 percent of the women who returned to work after childbirth did not have access to extended families to provide child-care, and the state made few provisions in this regard. Another survey (Straker et al., 1990) found that less than 1 percent of South Africa's more than 4 million black preschool children are cared for in child-care centers. The extent to which black parents are hard-pressed to provide adequate care for their children is clear. Although their earnings are vital for the survival of their children, their long working hours, including the time spent travelling over considerable distances, means that the children are often left in inadequate care for twelve or more hours each day (Wilson & Ramphele, 1989). Research has proven that adequate day care during the first five years of life can make a dramatic difference to children from disadvantaged environments, not only regarding their scholastic achievement, but also in the areas of prosocial behavior, self-regard and impulse control (Wilson & Ramphele, 1989). The negative consequences of failure to provide adequate child care—stunted physical, emotional and scholastic development—are well known, along with a growing incidence of child abuse, neglect and incest, teen pregnancy and substance abuse (Davie, 1990).

POVERTY

The expression *violence of poverty* can be seen as another kind of metaphorical violence (Degenaar, 1990). The word *violence* is used because poverty forces people to live a subhuman life. Because poverty can be perpetuated by political, social and economic structures, the violence of poverty is part of structural violence. While poverty forces people to live a subhuman life, economic structures can force poverty upon people. The central problem of today's world may be seen as the violence of poverty, which keeps over two-thirds of the world's population in a subhuman condition, the violence of revolt when peaceful demands have no effect, and the violence of repression with which the powerful try to crush the demands of the poor.

Approximately two-thirds of all black people in South Africa have to eke out a subsistence below the minimum living level. In the reserves or homelands the situation is even worse. The elderly and disabled, and women and children are the most vulnerable to the risks of destitution, starvation, and death due to the blows of fate that can destroy those who are already poor. Examples of the latter are droughts, seasonal famine, unemployment, forced resettlement and the effects of the worldwide recession (Wilson & Ramphele, 1989). In parts of South Africa the infant mortality rate for black children is unacceptably high, often caused by the ill-advised practice among young mothers who, wishing to be "modern," feed babies powdered milk (in insufficient quantities and using contaminated water) rather than use breast-feeding. Malnutrition and sickness among preschool children is especially serious in view of the finding that hunger at a young age can damage the growth of the brain and retard intellectual development. One-third of all black children up to the age of fourteen suffer from malnutrition. "But it is the famine of the mind and of the spirit which is perhaps even more serious" (Wilson & Ramphele, 1989, p. 175).

The constant and demoralizing economic worries about loss of jobs, income or homes and the associated feelings of insecurity and fear are just as real as the physical deprivations caused by poverty. Children are inevitably the victims when their caregivers are disempowered and alienated by the concomitants of poverty. The insecurities and fears experienced by those who are poor are often further exacerbated by alcohol—sometimes the only available form of relaxation (Wilson & Ramphele, 1989). Children not attending school also find solace in alcohol, as do women breast-feeding babies. The disruptive effect of the blossoming liquor trade in urban and rural areas on family life need not be belabored. Finally, in the words of David Hamburg (cited in Wilson & Ramphele, 1989):

> Poverty is partly a matter of income and partly a matter of human dignity. . . . Let us speak then of human impoverishment: low income plus harsh disrespect. . . . To speak of impoverishment in this sense is to speak of human degradation so profound as to undermine any reasonable and decent standard of human life. (P. 5)

ENVIRONMENTAL DEPRIVATION

Concomitants of poverty are bleak, stimulus-reduced surroundings and grinding boredom. In many small "dorps" or towns, and especially in the rural areas, there is virtually nothing to do. There are no fields to till and no cattle to tend. "Boredom hangs like a dark cloud. And, closely associated with it, despair" (Wilson & Ramphele, 1989).

Rural landscapes are often totally denuded of foliage. Every twig and rock has been used as firewood or to build shelter. Many township dwellings consisting of two or three tiny rooms still lack electricity and proper sanitation and may be shared by as many as ten to sixteen other persons.

Fifty years ago anthropologists reported on the rich traditional social structures with colorful rituals of kinship and neighborliness—these have all but disappeared. Hopelessness, poverty and changing values, together with poor educational background, have led parents to lose confidence in their ability to give direction, apply values and discipline, and indeed, communicate in any meaningful way with their children (Davie, 1990).

EXPOSURE TO CRIMINAL VIOLENCE

One of the most tangible social consequences of poverty is crime (Wilson & Ramphele, 1989). Where there is acute poverty, where work is difficult to find, and where society is in a process of upheaval, people are more likely to assault and to rob. Crime is both a product and a cause of the insecurity, misery and despair in which millions of South Africans find themselves trapped. The vulnerability of women and children living without male protection, especially in the densely crowded rural resettlement areas, is one of the hidden realities of life in South Africa. The Carnegie Commission provided one graphic description of how women in KwaZulu would lie in fear in their beds, while outside, the "tsotsis" (criminal gangs) would call out, "Is anybody at home?" If she should answer, or keep quiet, the gang would know that there was no man in the house. They would then break down the door and rob, assault or rape the women and children inside.

Because there are no parks or sports fields in many urban areas, the children are forced to play in filthy open lots and seek their own pastimes. Like children everywhere, they identify with and emulate the dominant characters of the neighborhood—the gangsters. In their games they reenact the sensational scenes they observe in the crime-ridden streets. Many communities in South Africa are plagued by instability, lawlessness and violence. For example, the Msinga area in northern Natal, where survival depends on an underground economy, is ridden with theft, poaching, interclan fighting, and the cultivation and sale of "dagga" (marijuana). Power is wielded by gangs of young men who have learned to live by illicit means and to impose their authority through the barrel of a gun. More guns find their way into the community from national servicemen who exchange them for "dagga." The violence in Msinga left at least 100 people dead in 1983 alone. The sense of fear and insecurity to which children are exposed every day of their lives is an especially insidious form of abuse. An alarming spread of gangsterism has been associated with devastating scenes of violence by children as young as six, who use knives, axes and pangas to butcher other children.

NEGLECT OF THE DISABLED

On a worldwide scale, an average of one in ten persons suffers from some kind of disability. In South Africa, the inadequate and fragmented nature of facilities for the disabled is a major problem (Wilson & Ramphele, 1989). Lack of services, especially for children, is a cause for grave concern. For example, in many communities there are no day-care services for mentally retarded children. The normal schools carry a disproportionate load of the day care. The most severely handicapped are most in need, as they cannot be accommodated in the schools. The subsistence provided by each person in a poor family is vital to survival. The presence of a noncontributing member, especially one who has special needs, necessitates the redistribution of resources such as education and nutrition, and may plunge the family into destitution. This is exacerbated when the disabled person is a child who cannot be left alone, and whose survival necessitates a potentially wage-earning adult to stay at home. The needs of disabled children living in the rural areas are likely to be even less well taken care of than those of disabled children in the metropolitan areas.

INADEQUATE HEALTH CARE

Despite the considerable natural resources of the country, hunger and poor nutrition are significant problems in many black households. Together with poor socioeconomic conditions, this weakens people's resistance to illness. Diseases of poverty, such as gastroenteritis and tuberculosis, are endemic. Some 33 percent of black children are stunted for their age, and black children are fourteen or fifteen times more likely to die before their fifth birthday than white children (Dowdall, 1990). Overall rates of nonnatural causes of death (homicide, suicide, motor vehicle accidents and unintentional injuries) among South African children are high compared to both developed and developing countries of the world. According to Kuhn (1990), nonnatural causes of death contributed to 64 percent of the deaths in white children between five and fourteen years in 1984. In the same year, 60 percent of Asian and colored and 38 percent of the deaths in black children were caused by nonnatural causes. Road accidents, drowning and homicide were the most prevalent nonnatural causes of death. Significantly, most of the motor-vehicle-accident-related deaths involved black children as pedestrians, while white children were mostly passengers. Nonfatal traumatic brain injury is much more common in African and colored children than in whites. However, the way in which violence affects children's health is not simply through trauma. Stress-related illness and psychological effects need to be further investigated. Violence may also influence children's health by disrupting health care provision. Political violence has disrupted attendance at clinics and also the provision of basic services necessary for maintenance of health, such as water, sanitation, streetlighting and transport.

Infant mortality rates (IMRs) are particularly revealing when they are considered as robust measures of the overall health of populations. These rates are especially sensitive to social influences (Kuhn, 1990). The dramatic differences between the IMRs of the various population groups reflect the structural violence in a racially stratified society. The IMRs for whites tend to be about 12.4 per thousand, 17.9 for Asians, 51.9 for coloreds and between 94 and 124 for Africans. Diseases related to poverty, such as diarrhoea and measles, contribute to 50 percent of the deaths in African and colored children, while only 7 percent of the white deaths under the age of one year are caused by these factors. The rate of malnutrition-induced kwashiorkor and pellagra is disproportionately high among blacks (Straker et al., 1990). Periodic outbreaks of measles and polio—entirely preventable diseases—still kill hundreds of black children. Deaths due to diarrhoea should also be preventable through the provision of basic services, sufficient and pure water, sanitation, and safe food distribution. On a secondary level, simple oral rehydration therapy should have prevented most of these deaths due to diarrhoea.

The nutritional status of children in depressed rural areas is another sign of structural neglect. The immunization status of children is particularly poor in rural, homeland areas (Kuhn, 1990). A feature of urbanization has been the refusal to accommodate new arrivals in the city and the corresponding growth of the squatter fringe in periurban areas, often considered illegal and hence not provided with basic facilities. The IMRs are high in these informal settlements and also in villages "resettled" by way of forced removals, where IMRs may be twice as high as in established villages. According to Bentley and Miller (1990) children in resettlement areas tend to have heavy parasite infestation (schistosomiasis, hookworm and roundworm). The migrant labor system has contributed to infant death through the spread of sexually transmitted diseases, notably congenital syphilis and AIDS. Finally, gross inequality exists in the distribution of health services at all levels. Malnutrition is particularly prominent in some homeland areas where shortages of human resources, facilities and medicine are acute.

A LOST GENERATION?

A considerable volume of literature on responses of children to stress and abuse of various kinds has emerged over the last ten years in South Africa. Many have voiced concern regarding the brutalization of a generation of children—a generation bereft of the values of justice, democracy and caring for others. Indeed, earlier studies of children in stressful situations tended to assume that they are necessarily damaged, whereas more recent studies suggest that damage is by no means inevitable or irreversible (Dawes & Tredoux, 1990). Following theorists like Piaget and Vygotsky, reconceptualization of the issues in developmental theory has led away from what might be termed a main-effects model of development to an interactive model in which a multidimensional approach to development is postulated (Bentley & Miller, 1990). Social constructivist views explain how potentially stressful events are mediated by systems of meaning existent in the individual, in the family, and in the community. Stressors do not simply exist "out there." The events themselves are socially constructed, as are forms of response to events regarded as stressful. This approach negates the positivistic notion that stressors impact on individuals in automatic or predictable ways. Within the complex matrix made up of events, the child's personality, the family, the school and the social and political environments, it becomes difficult to isolate some variables as causes and others as effects. It is more useful to acknowledge an interactive process to account for all these factors, as well as for others. A linear model of cause and effect is inappropriate and misleading (Gibson, 1990).

The social constructivist approach should not be interpreted to imply that, because events and responses are socially mediated, the effects of exposure to violence are minimal (Dawes & Tredoux, 1990). What the approach does highlight is that the effects are likely to vary, depending on conventional understandings operating in conjunction with factors like the child's developmental level, temperament and the type of exposure. It is the balance between risk, stress and protective characteristics in the child and his/her care-giving environment that accounts for the wide variety in range of outcomes (Bentley & Miller, 1990). The constructivist approach explains why children do not have to be detained or assaulted in order to be affected by political violence, thus drawing our attention to the substantial majority of children who are simply growing up in an environment where structural violence exists (Gibson, 1990). The sequelae of growing up in a violent society are not limited to a clinical syndrome such as posttraumatic stress disorder. Children can also be affected in more subtle ways that involve their moral and political socialization.

Research shows that the warmth of the mother-child bond and the resilience of the mother may be an especially important mediating factor, tending to act as a buffer against the emotional distress of the child (Bentley & Miller, 1990). Also important is the child's perception of the events and the reasons for their occurrence. Dawes and Tredoux (1990) found that symptoms of emotional distress following exposure to political violence was related to age and sex, with a reduction of symptoms in adolescent boys. They ascribed this to the emergence of gender-specific norms of acceptable conduct under stress. It was also speculated that the boys had been exposed to the rhetoric of the struggle and political protest activities, which helped them to make sense of the events. Straker and associates (1990) add that the specific form the reaction may take is heavily influenced by meanings ascribed to the stressor, the social demand characteristics of the situation, and the survival value of particular forms of expression. The latter two factors differ according to whether stress is historic or current—for example, aggression has a survival value in a war situation, while in peace it is counterproductive.

The degree to which involvement in political violence can be construed in heroic terms seems to be an important mediator of the individual's reaction. This is confirmed by Straker and colleagues (1990), who found that older children saw a police invasion and being arrested as an affirmation of their status as freedom fighters, thus raising their self-esteem and offsetting the negative impact of the traumatic events. Younger children are less likely to have this sort of ideological support, which might contain stress reactions. Witnessing the death of a vigilante was not significantly stressful for either the younger or the older children observed by Straker and her cocounselors. This death was seen as legitimate—just retribution for a previous murder and because the victim was defined as an enemy of the liberation struggle. This distressing finding confirms studies of Vietnam War veterans in which it was found that the ability to dehumanize the enemy affected the soldiers' responses to combat exposure and abusive violence (Straker et al., 1990).

Dowdall (1990) confirms the social constructivist view. Because the detainees he studied were individuals with different histories, support systems, vulnerabilities and resilience, they responded differently to the experience of detention. Some were strengthened in their resolve and commitment to the struggle, while others were profoundly damaged. Their social and political groupings and their construction of the detention experience—how they made sense of it—were important determinants. Specifically, the presence of a political and organizational support network and a coherent ideological way of making sense of the experience serve as important buffers against possible confusion and demoralization as a result of the abuse. Indeed, detention—intended to intimidate and demoralize—sometimes had the unintended consequence of politicizing and activating previously apathetic and uninvolved children and families.

In the study by Dawes and Tredoux (1990) it was found that while some children no doubt emerged from the experience of violence with hardened attitudes and talk of killing and hatred, this was not the uniform response. Many children expressed a wish to forgive their attackers and to explain the incorrectness of their behavior. In a South Africa where the killing continues, it is indeed an open question: What has to happen before the mold of conventional notions of forgiveness and morality break down?

CONCLUSION

Researchers and practitioners who work with damaged children should use all the power at their disposal to improve our understanding of development under adverse conditions, and to advance our ability to intervene so as to prevent and reduce risk in children's lives (Donald & Dawes, 1994). Interventions should seek to change those factors promoting vulnerability, while those promoting resilience should be fostered.

In the opinion of Ramphele (1994), South Africa's history has been characterized by the nation's failure to nurture its children. What is now needed is nurturance and support for the youth. Ramphele echoes Straker by saying that the degree to which proper nurturance and care can be provided for children, and the degree to which they are socialized towards tolerance, will determine the extent to which South African youth can be transformed from faces in a revolution to whole persons in a peaceful world.

9

Adolescence in a Changing Society

South Africa is a society in the throes of major and rapid sociopolitical change. Many societies have experienced large historical upheavals, but Burman (1986) argues that the scale and combination of forces such as urbanization, mass immigration and detribalization in conjunction with the effects of social engineering measures such as mass population removals and influx control, plus political unrest, places South Africa very high on the list of societies in the midst of fundamental societal change. At the same time, the age distribution of the African population is taking on an increasingly "pyramidal" shape, with the proportion of younger people in a constantly growing relation to the proportion of older people. It is estimated that about 45.5 percent of the total African population is under twenty (Hyslop, 1990). The sheer number of youth in society has put them at the center of the crisis in South Africa.

CONTRADICTORY DEFINITIONS OF CHILDHOOD

Divergent and contradictory definitions of childhood and adolescence exist not only in the legal system—where state maintenance for African children stops when they turn sixteen, while white and colored children are eligible for state support up to the age of eighteen—but also between the different cultural groups. A Jewish boy becomes classified as an adult—but only in a circumscribed religious sense—after his bar mitzvah at the age of thirteen. Boys who have undergone initiation ceremonies in certain African communities are regarded as men within those societies and may no longer be disciplined by women, irrespective of their age. Boys are usually initiated during the early teens, but they may be as young as six (Burman, 1986). The implications of the ambiguous status of these individuals in the socialization of male children, where the number of female-headed households is increasing alarmingly, are disconcerting. These "adult men," however, may remain in school, where they have the status of "children" and "scholars." Many of these "scholars" are economically dependent on the family up to and even beyond the age of twenty-five due to high failure rates and the slim prospects of dropouts finding employment. When the Department of Education and Training gazetted new regulations to restrict the admission of eleventh and twelfth grade students over the age of twenty, eighth, ninth and tenth grade students over the age of eighteen, and primary pupils over the age of sixteen, it was commented that there could be serious social consequences, as the age ruling would turn thousands of young people onto the streets in a period of severe unemployment (Samuel, 1990). This phenomenon of disturbed age system among black youths raises several issues, the first question being, How do present patterns relate to older, traditional patterns?

DISTURBED AGE-SET DYNAMICS

Accounts of age systems within societies stress the dynamics of horizontal unity and vertical subordination (Spencer, 1990). The dominance of the elders is achieved by cultivating the charismatic aspects of middle and old age. The equality of age-mates creates a close fellowship or communitas—a peer bond that cuts across rivalries in other spheres of existence. Fairly rigid formal stratification by age, such as is commonly found in traditional African cultures, resembles the societal groupings created by kinship and marriage (Mayer & Mayer, 1990). Whereas formal systems of kinship are widely recognized as important structural characteristics of society, there has been little recognition of the structural importance of age systems. Viewing adolescence in South Africa within a framework of age-sets seen as interactive social systems, is illuminating.

In the context of age-set dynamics, some forms of animal social organization have intriguing parallels with human society, where full adulthood is similarly bounded by the marginal phases of adolescence and old age, especially among males: those that have difficulty entering the arena and those that are edged out. Spencer (1990) tells how on an African safari, his Samburu guide drew his attention to two herds of gazelle. The guide, projecting the rudimentary organization of his own society, explained that the one herd consisted of the "elder" and his "wives," while the other, in which several gazelle frisked with one another, was the herd of the young "warriors" who had been excluded from the parent herd. This kind of social organization, in which young males in their physical prime are kept subordinate by physically weaker, but morally superior older males, might be taken as an illustration of the shift from "nature" to "culture" if one were to indulge for a moment in evolutionary speculation. Following this line of argument, one might see a movement from the most rudimentary forms of community life as a shift in emphasis between different forms of power: from brute physical prowess to "status," culminating, in more advanced societies, in power being distributed by "contract." Obviously, these shifts have profound implications for the balance of power between the younger and the older age-sets within a society.

Transactional approaches to the relations between age-sets are concerned with the inequalities and opportunities associated with the generations. The jostling for power between age-sets in various cultural settings has been the focus of fascinating studies. Gulliver's work (Spencer, 1990) revealed the rich cultural overlays and the symbolic interactions built around the dynamic shifts in the balance of power between age-sets. This is seldom a "comfortably harmonious affair" (Spencer, 1990)—a statement borne out by Philip and Iona Mayer's account of the traditional patterns of adolescence among Red Xhosa boys in South Africa.

Traditionally, Red Xhosa youth organizations were peripheral to the adult community, where they were tolerated—on pain of physical punishment—only in so far as they did not impinge on adult affairs (Mayer & Mayer, 1990). At their own gatherings, these adolescents (Mtshotsho) competed for status with increasing violence by "playing sticks" or cudgel duels. Significantly, their initiation was in the hands of senior elders and occurred at the critical period when this violence threatened to get out of hand. After initiation (undergone most commonly at an age between eighteen and twenty-three), they transferred to the much more sedate organizations made up of young men (Intlombe) who had already distanced themselves from the raucous fights of the boyhood groups, cultivating values (such as public speaking, debate and wise judgment) important for eventually achieving status as elders. The most crucial aspect of training boys into manhood was to get them to give up force and commit themselves instead to the rule of law (*umthetho*) and respect (*imbeko*). This transformation from "nature" to "culture" was perceived by the Xhosa society as a change from "bush" to "homestead," from "quasi-animal" to "human," eventually qualifying these young men to take up adult responsibilities.

In contrast to the Intlombe, where force and violence were abhorred, in the Mtshotsho, conflict was handled by the use of force. Law itself was something that had to be enforced by blows. Battles (*amadabi*) were mass confrontations between Mtshotsho groups from different regions. Although these boys did not use knives as did fighting gangs in town, the definition of "stick" or "cudgel" was stretched to include knobkerries, sharp, pointed sticks and sometimes even battle-axes and sharpened picks. From colonial times, local adults, assisted by white magistrates or black chiefs, have attempted to suppress some of the Mtshotsho's activities, notably the unsupervised mingling of the sexes during parties and the physical dangers posed by fighting with dangerous weapons. Chiefs and headmen constantly issued prohibitions against carrying dangerous weapons, to no avail.

It must be noted here that warfare has been prominent in Xhosa history. Intercommunal fighting and, especially, a series of wars against colonial aggression takes up much of the late eighteenth and early nineteenth centuries. Young men were the nation's warriors, and initiation was a step up in military as much as civil status, entitling them to own the adult weapon—the lethal spear. As part of the colonial pacification after conquest, the obligation of the initiated young men to become soldiers was replaced by an obligation to renounce fighting. However, the traditional Red Xhosa society—not having been exposed to Christian mission ideologies—did not take kindly to enforced pacification and disarmament. The public insistence on the unmanliness of fighting might be suspected of covering ambivalent attitudes (Mayer & Mayer, 1990). Although dignity forbade grown men from attending boys' fights and battles, tacit condonation was expressed by defining boys as "irresponsible" and "hard to control," thus enabling elders to draw vicarious satisfaction from the fighting without appearing to be compromised themselves. By saying that there was no way to stop them, the elders were representing the boys as the one remaining pocket to have defied pacification "perhaps even a kind of shadow fighting arm in succession to the vanished spearmen of former times" (Mayer & Mayer, 1990, p. 43). Within the context of contemporary intergroup violence in Natal's rural tribal districts and the seemingly endless bloodletting in the urban ghettoes, these speculations have a chilling ring of truth.

INTERGENERATIONAL TRANSFER OF KNOWLEDGE AND RESOURCES

Taking up Spencer's (1990) account, ritual knowledge in traditional societies is often a relatively closed system of beliefs that provides the idiom in which the authority of older people is couched. Numerous cross-cultural studies have emphasized the importance of the control of information and resources for accumulating and maintaining prestige and power among the elderly. The elders in traditional African societies are seen as repositories of cultural understanding, their social networks and diplomatic skills as valuable community assets. The older generation has the task of transferring to the next generation the system of beliefs and the society's symbolic superstructure, maintaining power and dignity by their ability to interpret and give meaning to social existence.

In contrast to the open competition for power among the Arusha tribe of Africa (Gulliver in Spencer, 1990), an alternative model is the manipulation of knowledge. In this framework, what is concealed may be more important than the knowledge itself. Gerontocratic organization based on a hierarchy of secrecy characterizes societies where older people hold control over symbolic beliefs. The Baktaman of Papua, New Guinea, and the Kpelle of Liberia are excellent examples, but this kind of social organization is probably characteristic of most societies that practice initiation ceremonies, often not immediately recognizable as such in more sophisticated Western guises. Academics may recognize with some chagrin that the following description of Kpelle secret societies might—without stretching the imagination too far—apply to a Western university:

The premise of knowledge placed the elders in the central arena and the premise of ignorance placed the youths on the periphery from where they had to buy their way in. However, the overall pattern was not one of elders passing on cultural traditions, but of withholding more than they taught in order to retain control over the young (Spencer, 1990, p. 9).

Older men played a prominent role in the Red Xhosa initiation ceremonies, where they would step forward and publicly harangue the silent novices. Mayer and Mayer (1990) observe that it is as if the task of taming the dangerous age and socializing it regarding violence and sexuality was more than could be left to the family and peer group who handled it for younger ages. It is easy to see that apart from an inevitable process of modernization, apartheid can be held largely responsible for upsetting the power balance in this typical African society by disempowering the older generation and discrediting the traditional knowledge they had to offer.

AMBIGUOUS STATUS AND POWER ROLES

To exemplify the ambiguous status and power roles in which an adolescent might be enmeshed, consider a fictitious case study. A young male of, say twenty-three years old, may, in terms of chronological age and Western standards, be a young adult—he may indeed be a parent himself—and in legal terms fully responsible since the age of twenty-one, yet be a financially dependent member of a female-headed household. Because he was only able to go to school for intermittent years when the family's limited funds allowed it, and may have failed once or twice, he might very well find himself in a tenth grade classroom, while the average age of white children in this standard would be fourteen to fifteen years. His ambiguous status would be further complicated if he were a "comrade," that is, a member of the youth brigade of the black liberation movement, because these groups have, in many instances, taken on a role of leadership and authority in communities where they have become the political voice and vanguard for an older generation hopelessly disempowered by apartheid. The future vision of alternative education implies a formalized recognition of a reconceptualization of age roles in the South African society—the young have staked a claim to full participation in the evolution of educational policy and practice (Gardiner, 1990a).

EROSION OF TRADITIONAL COMMUNITY STRUCTURES

If this hypothetical individual were living in a rural area, his status would be even further complicated by the position he occupies in the uneasy dichotomy between traditional tribal authority structures and the modern political groupings. Examples abound in which the authority of the tribal headman and his council, traditionally the domain of elderly men, has been successfully challenged by groups of comrades, many of them children by anyone's standards. This erosion of traditional community structures was of course indirectly caused by apartheid, as the tribal authorities were often seen to be mere puppets of the white regime, who propped them up as long as they remained docile. Also, in urban townships youth groups have usurped the authority usually wielded by more senior members of the community, often taking the lead in mass political actions. Like the Khmer Rouge children in Cambodia, "comrades" have instituted "people's courts" where they have tried and sentenced adults for crimes such as noncompliance with stay-aways.

As with other contemporary phenomena, it is useful to bear in mind the indigenous cultural roots of this phenomenon. In traditional Red Xhosa Intlombe (young men's social organizations), for example, their typical pursuit was to "discuss things" or "hear cases" (disputes between members) with adult-style oratory and formality (Mayer & Mayer, 1990). The Intlombe had several specially designated functionaries. The most important of these was the so-called "magistrate" (*iMantyi*), with special responsibilities in hearing cases. To become "magistrate" one had to excel at "speaking" or "persuading people." Although oversimplification is an ever-present danger, it is easy to see how apartheid's social engineering successes, coupled with the South African culture of intolerance and violence, may have contributed to the societal distortions that created "people's courts," where young comrades came to try and judge their elders, inflicting harsh punishments, not excluding execution by stoning or necklacing. The loss of confidence in the police, the cultural inappropriateness and the consequent rejection of apartheid's structures of justice, tainted by the fact that they enforced apartheid laws, were also contributory factors (Matshekga, 1991).

POLITICIZATION AND EMPOWERMENT OF YOUTH

Research done in the late 1960s by Geber and Newman (Foster, 1986) concerning the attitudes of nearly 1,000 adolescents from Soweto aged between seventeen and eighteen showed that developmental processes may coalesce into three major attitudinal structures: radical, accommodatory, or resigned-apathetic-alienated. The accommodated group displayed a conservative set of attitudes, endorsing traditional support of church and tribal affiliations, and acceptance of the wider political system. This group was optimistic about the educational system as a means for solving personal and social needs. The radical group rejected both tribal and political institutions, expressing doubt about the educational system as a means to achieve personal aspirations. This group also preferred the English language and showed a high degree of cognitive complexity in their responses. Although they evidenced positive views of personal and family relationships, they felt resistance toward formal authorities. The resigned group evidenced a depressed and resigned set of attitudes, with acceptance of the political and tribal status quo. This attitude appeared to be based on a belief that there were no choices. The latter group displayed generally low levels of personal and social aspiration accompanied by high levels of hostility and criminality, as evidenced in a projective personality test. These three attitudinal positions denote very different intergroup strategies, and evidence of the past decade clearly shows the radical strategy to be dominant among black youth.

The Congress of South African Students (COSAS) was the largest of the student organizations reflecting the dramatic mobilization and organization of youth since the seventies. By the end of 1984, it was estimated that well over 500,000 students had been involved in protests against the education system. The issues were the age-limit regulations, lack of democratic representation, excessive corporal punishment and sexual abuse of students by teachers—all of these clearly related to the education system. However, students increasingly linked their educational grievances to wider community and political issues, such as the withdrawal of the police and military from the townships, the resignation of community councelors, a reduction in rents and the reinstatement of dismissed workers (Samuel, 1990).

The politicization and empowerment of black youth have certainly been one of those inevitable, unforeseen spin-offs of a massive social engineering project. Simply put, the youth occupied the societal power vacuum created by the political and human disempowerment of the older generation. Mayer and Mayer's (1990) account of traditional Xhosa youth organizations reveal that Intlombe groups typically engaged in "hearing cases" concerning disputes between members in regard to breaches of the seniority etiquettes governing relations between age groups. The youth organizations formed a marginal category—the autonomy they enjoyed from the adult world was "in a sense a *quid pro quo* for their noninterference in it, and for not troubling adults with their sexuality, fights or problems" (Mayer & Mayer, 1990, p. 40). Their "courts" were held in disused or borrowed huts or out in the veld, and in adult terms, the "magistrate" of the Intlombe had no real domestic, political, legal or ritual power. The extradomestic and extracommunity nature of these youth courts has been dramatically reversed in its modern township manifestation, where many have been tried and sentenced to brutal punishment or death. The long-term effects on these youngsters and on society at large when children "jump" a generation and find themselves in adult roles for which they may be cognitively and morally ill prepared, remains to be seen. At any rate, the dramatic events in South Africa shed some light on the universal interface between cultural and social factors in determining the real and symbolic boundaries between childhood and adulthood.

PREMATURE PARENTHOOD

If the fictitious case study mentioned previously concerned a female, her situation might be even further complicated by premature motherhood. Possibly she has been catapulted into parenthood by an abusing adult, or even inspired to reproduce by misguided political slogans calling on women to contribute to the struggle by swelling the numbers of blacks. Consequently, a girl of fourteen might be a mother, although barely literate and living with her own mother or grandmother in a multigenerational, female-headed home. Defining childhood as the period from birth to reproduction would imply that she has attained adulthood without passing through adolescence at all. Often her younger siblings are the same age or even younger than her own children, with intergenerational boundaries blurring. Also, being a female in a male-dominated society, and moreover, a black female in a society where women have, until recently, been afforded status and power hardly above that of a child, this child-mother's situation is one riddled with ambiguity and potential conflicts.

CONTEXTUALIZED ROLE DEFINITIONS

Due to the rapid sociopolitical change in South Africa, roles and characteristics of childhood, adolescence and adulthood have to be defined in highly contextualized terms. A person may be a child in the context of the family as an economic unit and also in the classroom where he or she is a pupil in need of educational assistance, be an adolescent in terms of psychosexual and cognitive development similar to peers in Western industrial settings, yet be incomparably more adult in terms of political consciousness and sophistication than adolescents in white affluent communities, who still have to be prodded toward responsible citizenship and a social conscience.

LACK OF ADULT ROLE MODELS

Hyslop (1990) suggests that the changing numerical balance between the generations has played a part in the undermining of parental authority, which has been a feature of recent times.

In a situation characterized by dramatic discontinuities between the experience of children and their parents or grandparents, the younger generation is robbed of the role models so essential for the transmission of values and experience that they have found useful for dealing with their world (Burman, 1986). For example, the transition from rural farming community to camp slum, as a result of forced removal and resettlement of entire communities (Roux in Burman, 1986), may render the accumulated expertise of the adult useless and, thus, liable to be rejected by the younger generation.

Changes in occupation and income can have much the same effect, albeit on a lesser scale. This phenomenon, which occurred a generation earlier for many Jewish and Afrikaans children, is illustrated in Buijs's contribution in Burman's book (1986), describing the experience of Indian children at a sugar mill in Natal. The same effects are achieved through rapid urbanization and the effects of apartheid, which may disrupt family life to such an extent that old values and behavioral norms can no longer serve for survival purposes. The normal role model, especially the male model, may also be removed by family breakup.

LACK OF MALE ROLE MODELS

The proliferation of violence involving youths may at least partly be explained by the concept of compensatory machismo. The suggestion is that in a society where female-headed households predominate and where masculinity is no longer achieved through initiation ceremonies or other institutionalized practices, adolescent males will try, on their own, to assert their masculinity. Where child rearing is assigned primarily to mothers, and where fathers are largely absent during boys' childhood, cross-sexual identity may result. This, in turn, must be undone by displays of "manly behavior traits." The resultant aggression is not rooted in anger, but in a felt need to escape from womanliness and to mark one's masculine gender (Segall et al., 1991).

INCREASED IMPORTANCE OF THE PEER GROUP

According to Spencer (1990) the notion of communitas—the bond of fellowship among peers—is intimately bound to the existence of group initiation ceremonies. Mayer and Mayer (1990) describe this phenomenon in Red Xhosa youth organizations, where the youths were taught to love each other. Late in life, many were still great friends with those they had met at the Intlombe. In the case of modernized urban black youth, the mental and physical ordeals of traditional initiations might be said to have been replaced by the shared experience of apartheid society and Bantu education. Although the forces of gerontocratic oppression have been replaced by the forces of racist oppression, the effect may be the same: The youth are drawn together as mere mortals, with a prevailing emphasis on total equality, sharing everything as a group, reduced to a uniform condition that transcends all distinctions of rank, kinship and wealth.

In a study conducted in the early 1980s, Kotze and Norval (Foster, 1986) found that parental influence upon the political socialization of black adolescents was minimal. In contrast to white adolescents, black matric pupils in the Johannesburg area were more substantially influenced by their peers in the development of political attitudes than by either parents or teachers. This was confirmed by Geber and Newman's 1980 study (Foster, 1986), in which it was found that the influence of the family upon the general attitudes and aspirations of Soweto high school pupils was considerably less pronounced than the familial influence reported in British and American literature. Dreyer's study of Zulu adolescents similarly reported large-scale rejection of parental values and norms.

EXPOSURE TO AND PARTICIPATION IN VIOLENCE

When the educational crisis erupted in the townships, scores were settled with collaborating teachers, schools were set afire and, taking to the streets, sticks were sharpened at both ends to enforce alternative education and people's courts. Authority was confronted head-on in the ghettos, flesh was lashed from collaborating buttocks with whips, and broken bottles were rammed up mouths of informing wombs. The resulting melee was then set afire with kicks and sticks and stones (Saayman, 1990).

The effects of psychological violence may be no less damaging than those of physical violence. Violating the dignity of a person means that he/she is not allowed to exercise his/her freedom of will (Degenaar, 1990). This violation is an assault on the integrity of the person, or it might imply restricting the person in the free development of his/her personality by an external power. Structural violence has also taken a heavy toll, with laws that created a structure curbing the freedom of the subjects unfairly or discriminating unjustly against certain persons, preventing them from attaining full citizenship.

CHANGING GENDER ROLES

McFadden (1990) points out that it cannot be assumed that because one is a member of a liberation movement dedicated to freedom and democracy, that one will be rid of sexism and misogynist attitudes. To fight for democracy at a general level, and have an unequal, repressive or even abusive relationship with a girlfriend, is not unheard of among the male freedom fighters. Teenage pregnancy and the abuse of women by boyfriends are related to the patriarchy of traditional African culture. When young women prefer to have a baby out of marriage, or seek marriage because they think it will give them status and privilege in the community, it shows serious problems of self-identity and dependence. There is a need to redefine the meaning of motherhood, parenting, womanhood, self-definition and male-female relations. Liberation education might have a dramatic impact on the education of women. At the Solomon Mahlange Freedom College for exiled youths in Tanzania, subjects have been reprioritized so that the hard sciences are at the top of the list and homemaking subjects, like domestic sciences, are absent. Women students are encouraged to take subjects such as physics, math and chemistry. Surprisingly, while the female students are in the hard science courses, many male students tend to prefer the social sciences, explaining that the social sciences are closer to politics, to political debate and decision making (McFadden, 1990).

ADOLESCENTS IN EXILE

Children in many situations in South Africa are forced to work out their own destinies. They have to seek or create their own values and lifestyles to an extent far greater than is usual in more settled societies (Burman, 1986). An extreme example is that of the youth activists who left the country in the decades since the 1976 uprising. McFadden (1990) describes the situation of the children at the Solomon Mahlange Freedom College in the Morogoro district of Tanzania, 1,500 miles from South Africa. The secondary school accommodated 350 students in 1989, their ages ranging between thirteen and twenty-three years. Problems of discipline and authority were the most difficult in exile communities, where most of the youths had no family member present. The responsibility of parenting was shouldered by the leadership in the community. Students were assigned to foster parents who provided support and advice over the weekends. Yet the differences in attitude between the older generation of exiles who were educated under apartheid and subsequently received no alternative education, and the youth who received little else, caused intergenerational difficulties.

WASTED HUMAN POTENTIAL

The alarming drop-out rates among African and colored pupils reflect an enormous waste of human potential. In the early eighties about 46 percent of colored and 58 percent of African children dropped out of school after only four years (Pillay, 1990). Only 60.9 percent of a Sub A (first grade) group in 1972 reached Standard 2 (fourth grade) by 1975, meaning that two out of five pupils had not reached the fourth year of education and, in practice, would regress to almost complete illiteracy (Pillay, 1990, p. 36). In the same year, the Standard 5 (seventh grade) group consisted of 35.4 percent of the Sub A (first grade) group of 1969, indicating that nearly two-thirds of the pupils had not reached the seventh year of education, generally regarded as the minimum base for further education. Furthermore, of the pupils who first went to school in 1963, only 1.96 percent graduated from high school in 1975. By 1983, matters had further deteriorated due to the disruption in the schools—only 1.5 percent of the pupils in schools controlled by the Department of Education and Training reached matriculation (Pillay, 1990).

YOUTH UNEMPLOYMENT

High school enrollment ratios provide the ratio of pupils in secondary school to the population of "secondary school-going age." In this age-group, which may be taken as fifteen to nineteen, the percentage of African children enrolled in secondary school was 35 percent in 1980 (Pillay, 1990). This compares with nearly 90 percent of white children and 44 percent of colored children who were in school during the same period. The low high school enrollment ratios are a reflection of the high drop-out rate at the secondary level, where students often leave school to take up jobs to supplement the family income—if they can find employment. The white working population has had a monopoly on skilled jobs, while the vast majority of the black working population has been confined to semiskilled and unskilled jobs. Black school dropouts are prevented by insufficient and poor quality education from reaching high-level occupations. Furthermore, the black education system has failed to train school dropouts with marketable skills.

The school system has been ejecting hundreds of thousands of unqualified youths into a labor market in which their services are not in demand. Since the recent dramatic reforms in state education policy, rapidly growing numbers of black youths are entering a rapidly expanding school system. Yet upon exiting that system, they are faced with a stagnating labor market offering few opportunities. The sizeable group of teens and people in their early twenties who have not been able to break into the labor market has provided the social base of the youth movements outside the schools. A recent study cited by Hyslop (1990) indicated the desperation felt by both urban and rural African youths—they expressed considerably greater discontent over the lack of employment opportunities than they did over either political or educational grievances.

DISTORTED OR ARRESTED RACIAL-CULTURAL IDENTITY DEVELOPMENT

A study conducted during the 1960s by Lambert and Klineberg (Foster, 1986), which included a sample of 300 Zulu and Sotho children, found that African children aged six and ten referred to themselves primarily in terms of race. By age fourteen the most important self-descriptive category was gender, but race remained an important criterion. In comparison to children from eleven other countries, the African children were the only group for whom race was the most important self-description. This reflects the very real implications of the centrality of racial categorization and discrimination. Results consistently show that black children from an early age prefer white stimulus figures. On the forced-choice doll tests, three independent studies reported by Foster (1986) found a strong preference for the white doll figure among young black children. The white-preference results appear to be larger and more consistent than those reported in earlier American studies. Research using other techniques has provided further support for the phenomenon of out-group preference among black children.

Identification rather than preference indices are sometimes regarded as more significant. This is usually ascertained in the doll test by asking, "Show me the doll that looks like you." Misidentification (the choice of the white doll by black children) has been observed frequently among black children, especially among urban groups and girls, although there is a reduced incidence of misidentification in recent years (possibly owing to black consciousness ideology). Nevertheless, recent studies (Foster, 1986) suggest contradictory attitudes of black children toward their own group, with positive characteristics attributed to white figures and negative characteristics to black figures in a forced-choice test. The violence of overt suppression and detentions may have been only the tip of the iceberg when seen in the context of the massive structural violence of apartheid.

Gama (1990) reports the results of an opinion survey by the National Council of Mental Health. The following are some of the areas that young people experienced as stressful:

1. Lack of interpersonal skills was an important source of stress to the respondents, especially in the areas of communication, conflict resolution, problem solving, negotiation

and assertiveness. Interracial nonacceptance was mentioned, as was difficulty in communicating with parents, other adults and authority figures.

2. A lack of self-confidence was reported to have a negative impact on young people's self-regard and self-esteem. Social inequality and the rapid changes taking place in the country were mentioned as additional stressors.
3. Their inability to cope with and express emotions was another major problem.

The research cited above can only be regarded as indirect evidence, but it would not be unreasonable to propose that all these findings suggest disturbed, distorted or arrested racial-cultural identity development. Black identity development models are well represented in the one proposed by Sue and Sue (1990). The authors formulate a five-stage model summarizing the development that oppressed people experience as they struggle to understand themselves in terms of their own culture, the dominant culture, and the oppressive relationship between the two cultures. The five stages are: conformity; dissonance; resistance and immersion; introspection; and integrative awareness.

1. The conformity stage (also known as passive-acceptance or preencounter stage) is characterized by unequivocal preference for dominant cultural values and global racial self-hatred. The lifestyles, value systems and cultural as well as physical characteristics of whites are valued more than those of their own group. Because it has such a profoundly negative impact, this stage represents perhaps the most damning indictment of white racism.
2. During the dissonance stage the individual encounters information or experiences inconsistent with culturally held beliefs, attitudes and values, causing denial to break down and leading to a questioning and challenging of the attitudes and beliefs of the conformity stage. People generally move into this stage slowly, but a traumatic event may propel individuals into dissonance.
3. Resistance and immersion is a stage in which culturally different individuals tend to completely endorse their own group's views and completely reject the dominant group's values and culture as having no validity for him or her. Driven by guilt, shame, and anger, desire to eliminate oppression of the individual's group becomes a central motivation. Feelings of guilt and shame may be connected to a perception of having been a "sellout" in the past, while strong anger is directed at oppression, racism and the dominant group. Although this phase may be a natural reaction to an oppressive and discriminatory society, many South African youths may be entrapped in a stage that is basically a negative, and sometimes self-destructive, reaction against the dominant culture. The stance is not proactive and does not allow the individual to use all energies to discover who he or she is. Because self-definition is largely reactive (against white racism), positive self-definition in a proactive sense may be blocked. The individual may be required to submerge individual autonomy and individual thought in favor of the group goals.
4. Several factors may contribute in moving the individual to the introspection phase. The person may begin to feel that the intensity of feelings toward white society is psychologically draining and does not permit him/her to devote sufficient energy to self-

understanding or to his/her own racial-cultural group. Feelings of discontent and discomfort with rigidly resistant and immersive group views may be experienced, as well as concern with the blind ethnocentric rejection of other groups. There may be intense conflict between allegiance to their own group versus notions of personal independence and autonomy.

5. Persons who have attained the integrative awareness stage have developed an inner sense of security and can own and appreciate unique aspects of their own culture, as well as those of the dominant culture. Conflicts experienced in the previous stage are resolved, allowing greater individual control and flexibility. Acceptable and unacceptable aspects of all cultures are acknowledged, and all forms of oppression are rejected. A strong sense of pride in their own group does not imply that all group values are accepted unequivocally. Individual members of the dominant group may be trusted and liked. The constructive elements of the dominant culture are appreciated. White racism is seen as a sickness in society and white people as victims who are in need of help. The individual experiences a strong sense of self-worth and confidence. A high sense of autonomy is accompanied by an integrated self-concept that involves racial pride in identity and culture. The person can be bicultural or multicultural without a sense of having "sold out." The person perceives himself or herself as an autonomous individual who is unique (individual level of identity), a member of one's own racial-cultural group (group level of identity), a member of a larger society and a member of the human race (universal level of identity). One can only hope that the societal and educational forces in the "new" South African will be such that far greater numbers of youth attain this level of development than is presently possible.

CONCLUSION

Karl Mannheim's age-cohort theory (Spencer, 1990) brings together the notion of life stages and the problem of social change. Each generation in Mannheim's formulation is shaped by the impact of contemporary events. Successive generations fight different adversaries, both within and without. Each generation has a radically new contact with prevailing conditions that leads toward novel solutions. Contemporaries are seen to interact within a milieu that is different from that of their predecessors and they experience the same historical situation differently. In the course of aging, each cohort is uniquely marked by the imprint of history and leaves its own imprint. Victor Turner (Spencer, 1990), with his more symbolic approach to age-cohort theory in his concept of social dramas, has a bearing on adolescence in South Africa. Turner's concepts drew attention to the role of key figures at critical moments of their careers when they faced dilemmas that were symbolic of their time. Life crises in the lives of many South African youths cast them in the roles of martyrs, and were also key moments in South African history. According to Turner, key moments in history are also key transitions in the lives of all who partake in them and the symbolic trappings of the event itself, through the myth that grows around it, have the hallmarks of a rite of transition for society at large.

Part IV

Educational and Mental Health Issues

At present there is a "crisis" in psychology in South Africa. A mental health investigation has been initiated and a national task force appointed in order to reform the profession in all its aspects. These events are the result of a deep sense of unease about the mission, relevance and image of the profession and an awareness that mainstream psychology is irrelevant to the nature and needs of the majority black population. Presently, psychology in South Africa is at a crossroad. In chapters 10, 11, 12 and 13 the mental health needs of the majority black population are identified. Professional training programs for future psychologists, as well as the utilization of services and resources in delivery systems, are suggested. The psychologist's role in a divided and traumatized society is fully described. The issue of open schools and the need for multicultural skills for teachers, guidance specialists and other helping professionals in the school setting, are also explored. Guidance and counseling personnel, as well as social workers and psychologists, must not only be sensitized to racial and ethnic perspectives but must also be aware of approaches that are culturally encapsulated and ethnocentrically biased. A cross-cultural model for acquiring knowledge, awareness and skills is presented and guidelines for applying the cross-cultural model are given.

10

From Bantu Education to People's Education

Deep conflict over education is a major issue in the historical upheavals that have rocked South Africa in recent decades. Opposition to the segregated and inferior education for blacks in this country is not new, but since 1976, education has increasingly become an instrument of liberation, and schools the battlegrounds in the struggle for an equitable social order. The crisis is one of multiple inequalities and of ideological confrontation between apartheid and demands for equality and social justice. The education system has become a battleground of ideas over how to accomplish substantive economic and social changes in South Africa (Nasson & Samuel, 1990).

PREINDUSTRIAL EDUCATION

Keto (1990) makes the important point that if we define education as the transmission of a cultural heritage from one generation to another, then communities of indigenous South Africans had created effective formal and informal systems of traditional education before the Dutch arrived in South Africa to create a refreshment post in 1652. Whether this was done through initiation rituals or more informal means, there was always a congruent relationship between the training and the lifestyle young people encountered after "school." The society that controlled their education also determined their life chances once they had completed their "schooling." One may not today agree with which roles (e.g., gender roles) were assigned to people by these forms of education, but they did not socialize them for alienation. The arrival of the Europeans signalled the beginning of Western-style education, which sought to reflect and transmit the values, interests and priorities of Europe. For Africans, this kind of education meant the creation of discontinuities, for example, the acquisition of skills by young Africans that adult Africans often did not possess. "Education ceased to be coterminous with the experience of social life in the African community, became future-oriented and relied heavily on the vicarious experience described in books and explained by teachers" (Keto, 1990, p. 23).

THE MISSIONARY SCHOOLS

Religious institutions played a dominant role in the new education in South Africa. The earliest settlers, Dutch Calvinists, fostered functional literacy, since true believers were expected to read the Bible for themselves. Other colonial powers brought other denominations into the country. The roots of black education are, in many instances, traceable to the missionary schools established in the previous century. For example, in the Victoria East and Middledrift districts of the Ciskei, the great educational institutions like Lovedale (Presbyterian), St. Matthews (Anglican), and Healdtown (Methodist) took root in the middle of the nineteenth century. An analysis done when the Bantu Education Act of 1953 set up a separate department of education that took over and, in important instances, destroyed, the mission schools, found that virtually all school-age children in these two districts were in school at a time when, in South Africa as a whole, it was estimated that only one-third of African children between the ages of six and sixteen were in school (Wilson & Ramphele, 1989). The quality of education was good, albeit austere. One consequence of the mission schools in different parts of the country, and of the establishment, in 1916, of the university college of Fort Hare (which grew out of Lovedale), is the existence of a significant elite of educated black South Africans. After all, the Bible was published in Sotho, Tswana, Xhosa and Zulu a full fifty years before the first Afrikaans (as distinct from High Dutch) Bible was published.

BANTU EDUCATION AND CHRISTIAN NATIONAL EDUCATION

It was the same racially separatist philosophy espoused by the ruling National party that more than thirty years ago led to the creation of Christian National Education for whites and Bantu Education for blacks. Bantu Education was bitterly resented because government spokesmen made it clear that the policy was intended to ensure that blacks not be educated for jobs beyond their proper station in life, that is, menial laborers. In his notorious 1953 speeches to Parliament, Dr. H. F. Verwoerd spelled out that Bantu Education would create conditions for stabilizing a black urban underclass of semiskilled laborers. After 1959, Bantu Education would also provide a means of ideological incorporation of the bantustans or homelands and ensure the hegemony of the ruling class by entrenching a sense of national consciousness based on ethnicity and the illusion of self-determination (Cross & Chisholm, 1990). Undoubtedly, dramatic reforms since that time have resulted in more acceptable policies and improved facilities. Nevertheless, deep suspicion of the goals of Bantu Education remained. In 1990, Nkomo still describes apartheid education as, at best, "a policy of benign neglect, at worst, as a policy that promotes compulsory ignorance" (Nkomo, 1990, p. 295). This goes a long way toward explaining why, in 1976, children took to the streets, prepared to sacrifice their lives for the sake of educational reform.

DISPARITIES IN THE EDUCATIONAL STRUCTURE

African pupils, each with a subsidy of R234 in 1983–84, received only one-seventh (14%) of the subsidy of R 1 654 available for white pupils (Wilson & Ramphele, 1989, p. 141). These statistics understate the actual difference in subsidy to the two groups, as virtually all school-age white children are in school, while for black children, particularly in the rural areas, the proportion at school is well below the maximum. By 1980, virtually all (96%) white children were in school, while four out of every five (83%) Africans were officially estimated to be in school, although there is strong evidence to suggest that the latter is a considerable overestimate. If we combine the facts that expenditure per pupil and the proportion of children enrolled at school are lower for blacks than for whites, we find that state expenditure on education per head of population for blacks is one-tenth that for whites (Wilson & Ramphele, 1989). The following sections of this chapter set out the inadequacies and problems in the system of Bantu Education, which eventually caused the 1976 revolt and the creation of People's Education. Aspects that will be discussed include: limited access; poor quality; inadequate home support for learning; forced mainstreaming of children with severe handicaps; high failure and drop-out rates; inadequate tertiary educational opportunities; high rates of illiteracy coupled with limited employment prospects for those who have passed through the school system.

LIMITED ACCESS

Although some parts of the country have a fairly comprehensive network of schools, there is wide variation between areas. In some magisterial districts there are virtually no schools (Wilson & Ramphele, 1989). Even where schools exist, access is often hampered by limited transport facilities. Most children walk to school and the distances are often considerable.

One in five of all black South Africans lives on white-owned farms, which constitute about four-fifths of the land area of South Africa (Wilson & Ramphele, 1989, p. 146). Education on the farms is dependent on the existence of farm schools, and their existence is entirely at the discretion of the farmer, although the state does subsidize the school building and pays the teachers' salaries. The farm schools are invariably for primary levels only—few of them go beyond Standard 6 (eighth grade). Sending children to towns or cities to complete their education creates insurmountable difficulties for poor families, with few of them able to afford boarding fees. Consequently, few farm children have the opportunity of going to secondary school, thus ensuring that the next generation is also unqualified for any occupation other than underpaid farm labor. The real problem is that farm children are not getting the kind of education that will enable them to make the transition to urban jobs. At the same time, because of mechanization and the changing technology of production, the demand for unskilled labor is steadily shrinking. For many of these children, childhood ends between the ages of twelve and fourteen when the boys take their place alongside their fathers in the fields or in the white farmer's house and kitchen, if they are girls. Also, classrooms are not secure, as children are poached at peak harvest periods and sometimes removed to do intermittent work as herd boys or to perform other agricultural duties (Wilson & Ramphele, 1989).

LACK OF QUALITY

Although the proportion of children in school has risen rapidly over the last decade (by more than 7% per year), the failure of government to provide adequate resources to fund this expansion has meant that the quality of education provided has been abysmally low. This lack of quality, particularly in comparison with what is available for white pupils, is manifested in the differential provision of teachers. In 1984, the average pupil-teacher ratio was 19:1 for whites and 41:1 for Africans. The shortage is most serious in primary schools (Pillay, 1990). What this often means in practice is classes of ninety children or more, which is educationally impossible (Wilson & Ramphele, 1989). Since the beginning of the 1970s there has been considerable improvement in the situation. However, the magnitude of the needs was simply beyond the system's capacity. Nkomo (1990) suggested that the only possible way to solve this problem would be to eliminate the military budget and dismantle the costly apartheid bureaucratic apparatus.

In South Africa there is both a quantity and a quality deficiency of teachers. Perhaps worse than the actual lack of teachers has been the inadequate teacher training. Whereas in white schools all teachers are matriculated and most of them (97%) have professional teaching qualifications, the proportion of African teachers without matriculation in 1983 was two-thirds (69%). The pattern is a vicious cycle of poorly qualified teachers, producing poorly qualified pupils, who in turn go on to become poorly qualified teachers (Pillay, 1990). The problems of large classes and poorly qualified teachers are reinforced by the lack of facilities. The general situation is still chronic despite the fact that the state has built a number of solid schoolbuildings around the country. Classrooms are overcrowded, desks insufficient, playing fields inadequate, windows shattered, toilets broken and textbooks unavailable. Libraries, laboratories and modern teaching aids like overhead projectors and video machines are virtually unheard of (Wilson & Ramphele, 1989).

The focus of education has also been on passive and rote learning. The character of apartheid education has been such that it has produced individuals, both black and white, who have their intellectual horizons proscribed (Nkomo, 1990). The possibility of conceiving alternatives to the prevailing social system has been inhibited and the capacity for critical thinking blunted. An additional problem is the use of biased and racist syllabi. In the past, much of the information in textbooks portrayed the white man as superior and always doing things for the black man, while the black man was represented as dutiful and respectful, his chief concern in life being the good service of his master (Nasson & Samuel, 1990). The lack of proper teacher training is exacerbated by a loss of student morale. Of course there are many teachers who are dedicated and who perform educational miracles in the face of impossible odds, but the Carnegie Inquiry (Wilson & Ramphele, 1989) reported many instances of appalling breakdown in schools, with teachers often drunk, absent from work, and sometimes even assaulting or raping pupils. This loss of morale might be attributed to the frustration, powerlessness and anger of the disenfranchised. Schoolchildren physically attack teachers, as they are the nearest symbol of an authority they reject. Schools have been taken over by "comrades," and teachers subjected to intense humiliation. An Inter-School Manual put out by students in Cape Town carried an article deriding the "petty bourgeois attitudes" of teachers and calling them a "misfit lot condemned to the Sewage Tanks of Athlone. . . . Their sole concerns are their cheques, their bonds on houses, their cars" (Naidoo, 1990, p. 129). Caught between the government, which paid their salaries, and militant students, who despised them for having "sold out" to the system, teachers have often found solace in drink (Wilson & Ramphele, 1989). In contrast to whites, who systematically increased their local control over the decision-making process that determined policy regarding the education of their children, blacks have had little control over educational policies and little access to policy making (Keto, 1990).

INADEQUATE HOME SUPPORT FOR LEARNING

Half a century ago, white South Africa was shocked by the first Carnegie Commission's finding that many white children came to school too hungry to concentrate. While school-feeding schemes soon alleviated this situation, today it is the black children who come to school hungry. The fact that one-third of black children under the age of fourteen are malnourished and underweight for their age speaks for itself (Wilson & Ramphele, 1989).

The sheer cost of education from the family's point of view is often an insurmountable problem. Fees and levies, textbooks, and school uniforms are unaffordable when a family is already living near or under the poverty line. There is pressure on older children to leave school in order to work and contribute to the family's income. Schooling is often interrupted for a year or more and sometimes even terminated because there is no money. Educational failure is part of a cycle of poverty, social ineffectiveness and ignorance (Gwalla-Ogisi, 1990). In the rural areas children are often left in the care of grandmothers, while their parents work in the metropolitan centers. In the absence of creches or preschools, even in the urban areas, an older brother or sister is then taken out of school to help at home and to take care of the small children.

ENFORCED MAINSTREAMING

Because of the prevalence of poor living conditions and poor nutrition, the incidence of handicaps and health-related deficits among African children is abnormally high. Yet handicapped, mentally retarded and learning disabled children in African schools are mostly mainstreamed:

> Not because it is a terrific idea and state of the art innovative practice, nor because it is a practice deemed the best for handicapped children, but only because it is the only alternative. The issue becomes that of efficiency in educating all children who can afford to be in school, i.e., providing any setting at all for children (Gwalla-Ogisi, 1990, p. 276).

There are few examples of preventive or remedial services or efforts in South Africa for Africans. In addition, it becomes very difficult to accurately assess real learning or emotional deficits in contrast to policy-related and system-created delays, underdevelopment and underachievement.

FAILURE AND DROPOUT

Of every 100 children who started school in 1969, the number who had matriculated by the end of 1978 was only four. The comparative figure for whites was 69 (Wilson & Ramphele, 1989). Of all the African children who left school in 1982, more than half (53%) had gone no further than Standard 2 (fourth grade), one-quarter of them leaving school without even obtaining Sub A. Only 10 percent of school dropouts in that year reached Standards 9 or 10 (eleventh and twelfth grade). Although the number of African pupils passing Standard 10 (twelfth grade) increased fourteen times between 1970 and 1983, it is matric exemption (which gives access to university and hence to professional careers), which is significant. In 1978, whites (who then made up 15% of the population) still constituted three-quarters (74%) of all matric exemptions, while Africans (who constituted 73% of the population) made up 16 percent of the total. In that year, only 5,000 black pupils qualified for university. The percentage of African pupils with exemption actually decreased in certain areas during the early 1980s (Pillay, 1990).

"BUSH" UNIVERSITIES

The great majority of the students at university are white. The eleven black universities in South Africa cater to specific African ethnic groups and are mostly situated in the homelands, comprising modern brick and concrete clusters unexpectedly placed in a rural landscape—hence the name *bush* colleges. In 1984, only 21 percent of students attending university were Africans, although they represented 73.5 percent of the population. Blacks are grossly underrepresented or nonexistent in such areas as engineering, architecture, astronomy, physics, food science and physiotherapy, to name but a few. This situation may be traced back to the recommendation of the Holloway Commission in 1954, that in the context of separate development, no courses should be offered in the African universities for which employment opportunities did not exist within their "own societies" (Nkomo, 1990). The universities have often been victims of bantustan bureaucracies and incongruously staffed and managed by conservative Afrikaner academics (Naidoo, 1990). Most of the university teachers are white. An important task of the black universities, as formulated by Commissioner J. H. Snyman (cited in Nkomo, 1990) while investigating student unrest at the University of the North, was to dissuade the educated blacks from being influenced by "subversive organizations." The alarmingly low number of Africans getting advanced technical education at the three technicons allocated them, completes the picture of inadequate tertiary education (Pillay, 1990).

ILLITERACY

In the context of what has been described thus far concerning the inadequacy of education for the majority of South Africans, the prevalence of illiteracy is not surprising. However, for a country whose industrial revolution has been under way for a full century and where more than half the population is urbanized, the degree of illiteracy in South Africa is still staggering (Wilson & Ramphele, 1989). According to the 1980 census, 33 percent of those Africans over the age of fifteen who completed the census form judged themselves to be illiterate, while 30 percent of those older than twenty had not achieved an educational level as high as Standard 4 (six years of schooling) and so were functionally illiterate. Among whites, by contrast, less than 1 percent assessed themselves to be illiterate, and the proportion older than twenty with less than Standard 4 education was only 2 percent. Those classified as colored or Asian fell, as usual, somewhere between Africans and whites. According to some estimates, the total number of illiterate adult Africans in South Africa is in excess of 4 million (Pillay, 1990). While the general level of education of the population as a whole may be improving, the number of young illiterates between the ages of ten and twenty-four, is highly disturbing, and may be as high as 3 million. In one rural district, Nkandla in KwaZulu, more than one-third of teenagers in the district had never been to school (Wilson & Ramphele, 1989).

Any well-educated urban dweller who has tried to milk a cow or to track game and shoot it for the pot can testify that the ability to read and write is not necessarily the most useful economic skill in some circumstances. But in a modern industrial economy it is difficult, especially in urban areas, to earn one's living without being literate, especially if jobs are scarce and employers make literacy the first criterion for selection (Wilson & Ramphele, 1989). A major need in South Africa is that of full educational opportunity for all, education that is relevant to the demands of the labor market.

LIMITED EMPLOYMENT PROSPECTS

It is the bleak economic environment in which school dropouts, half of them not even properly literate, find themselves when they leave school, that poses the most fundamental educational problem of all (Wilson & Ramphele, 1989). Unemployment is rife and getting worse, especially among black women and black school dropouts. A combination of factors interact to nullify the efficacy of education in gaining employment. Factors such as age, gender and, especially, contacts who are already employed, are better predictors of success than education. Employers have put at least some of the blame for stagnant productivity and falling profitability on the failure of the education system to adapt to the increasingly complex skill requirements of the industrial labor market (Nasson, 1990). Whatever the causes, a situation in which education no longer operates as a "giver of life-chances," except for a few, and in which one student in ten manages to pass ten years of schooling, is bound to cause massive dissatisfaction. Many young people have inevitably come to the conclusion that the current education system is worthless. The following sections of this chapter deal with the inevitable revolt against a system that has failed and the events following the disruption of schooling since 1976.

THE 1976 REVOLT

Up to the mid-1960s, the state put little effort into improving black secondary schools. In fact, there was a deliberate attempt to retard the growth of black urban secondary schools, so as to stem the tide of urbanization (Hyslop, 1990). In the early 1970s, the government moved to a more pragmatic interpretation of apartheid and the expansion of urban secondary schools was permitted in response to industry's increasingly complex labor needs. The result was that between 1970 and 1976 secondary enrollment more than tripled. By drawing the mass of urban youths into a common, oppressive and underresourced educational school system, Bantu Education had ironically provided a shared experience that unified them into a cohesive force (Cross & Chisholm, 1990). Instead of socializing students into tamely accepting the burdens of educational and other forms of inequality, black schooling rolled forward to become the "Trojan horse" within the apartheid state (Nasson, 1990). The huge disruption in black education was sparked in 1976 by new regulations stipulating that Afrikaans was to be made the medium of instruction for half of the high school subjects. Teachers and children felt that high failure rates were already caused by the existing requirement that mathematics and social sciences were examined in Afrikaans. Many felt that having to learn more Afrikaans, the language of the oppressor, would further restrict their capacity to find out about the world. After negotiations failed, pupils at Orlando West Junior School in Soweto went on strike. Other schools followed suit in the ensuing weeks. On June 16, 1976, Soweto pupils marched to the Orlando stadium. The huge protest march was broken up by police gunfire (Nasson & Samuel, 1990). The children won a moral victory, but in the process they incurred the armed wrath of the state.

Boycotts became more frequent and more violent and were sometimes joined by stay-aways (strikes) by workers. The violent reaction of the state—using whips, tear gas, rubber bullets, live ammunition, detention and sometimes torture—combined with the student unrest to create an intensifying spiral of violence. During the 1976 protest, several hundred children were shot and killed. During 1985 and 1986, the cycle of violence took on a ghastly pattern: Schoolchildren were shot during protest marches, thousands of protesters then marched to their funerals, the police took action, and more deaths resulted. After examining the evidence, the New York–based Lawyer's Committee for Human Rights described the process as a "war against children" (Wilson & Ramphele, 1989).

The slogan *liberation before education* was, in retrospect, based on a too-facile assumption that boycotting the school system would necessarily bring about a speedy end to the political system. Nevertheless, the revolt that began as a spontaneous uprising had political repercussions far beyond its time and region (Cross & Chisholm, 1990). It stimulated organization inside the country, among and beyond the student body, and sent many into exile in search of military training outside the country's borders. The painstaking task of grassroots organization around labor, health, community and educational issues was taken up. As the struggle continued, there were significant changes in organization, consciousness and strategy. The 1980 school boycotts demonstrated a marked sophistication. Democratic forms of school-based organization were explored, and acute analytical attention was given to the relation of schools to the capitalist economic system (Cross & Chisholm, 1990).

STATE RESPONSE TO THE CRISIS

In 1980, a new statute, the Education and Training Act, replaced the Bantu Education Act of 1953. This statute moved toward free and compulsory education, with more active involvement of parents and communities, and represented an attempt by the state to resolve the crisis. A modernized idiom of educational practice within a reform framework of equality was constructed (Nasson, 1990). Inspired by the recommendations contained in the 1981 De Lange Report, a massive attempt was made to wipe out the stigma of discriminatory apartheid education. The 1986–1987 percentage increases over 1985–1986 in per capita pupil expenditure amounted to 22 percent for Africans, 8 percent for coloreds and 30 percent for Indians. Significantly, expenditure for whites actually decreased by 5 percent in the same period. Total budget expenditure on African education for 1987–1988 reflected an annual increase of approximately 31 percent (Nasson, 1990).

The ruling Nationalist party paid for these reforms in terms of lost support by the blue-collar white Right, aggrieved at losing a customary privilege as scarce resources were being shifted away from white education. In addition, the reforms were viewed in a critical light by those who were supposed to benefit from them. Many perceived the reforms to be more discourse than actual educational provision (Christie, 1990). Others felt that they did not go nearly far enough. The restructuring of black education was seen to be inspired by self-interest on the part of the white government. It was as if the state, by upgrading black education, could address the problem of a white skilled labor shortage and at the same time provide greater educational opportunities to blacks in the urban areas. Accordingly, they could arrest the political ferment, as well as achieve their co-optive strategy aimed at the fusion of blacks into the ranks of the privileged middle class (Nkomo, 1990). Nasson (1990) sums it up by saying that the state's attempt to legitimize that which continues to be illegitimate did not succeed in winning mass support. Moreover, education forms a crucial popular base in the war of position being waged in South African politics.

PEOPLE'S EDUCATION

The failure of the state's education policy was heightened by the emergence of the black trade-union movement, the spread of black consciousness ideology, a significant downturn in the economy, the growing rate of unemployment and the political impact of the liberation of Angola and Mozambique (Samuel, 1990). By 1985 it became clear, however, that permanent boycotts made students increasingly difficult to organize and that immediate social transformations were not being achieved. Students were beginning to act autonomously from other sectors of the community, often in violent and arbitrary ways (Hyslop, 1990). This led to divisions between students on the one side, and parents, workers and teachers on the other. Teachers were often seen by the students as working for the system and were consequently humiliated or even attacked. The People's Education movement was an attempt to overcome these divisions. In October 1985, the Soweto Parents' Crisis Committee was formed to bring about unity of parents, students and teachers. At the subsequent founding conference of the National Education Crisis Committee in December 1985, the "Liberation Now, Education Later" approach was repudiated and replaced by a new strategy: "People's Education for People's Power" (Hyslop, 1990). This strategy signified that students would struggle for education from within the system, rather than withdrawing from it.

Within the context of People's Education, the arguments being advanced for the full participation of the young—by way of parent-teacher-student associations (PTSAs) and student representative councils—in the learning process, in classroom management and in curriculum design, is not a belated plea for child-centered, permissive or progressive education (Gardiner, 1990a). The transformation from passive and rote learning to creative participation was central to the concept of People's Education. Alternative education is, however, not limited to formal education. The radical reconceptualization of the nature of the school itself, and its relation to the community, presupposes a broader understanding of education in people's lives (Gardiner, 1990a).

Integral to the culture of opposition that was sparked by the children's uprising was the reconceptualization of people as national, not ethnic, subjects, and as belonging to a unified South Africa, not to fragmented ethnic units (Cross & Chisholm, 1990). An important recent development in this culture is the commitment to a search for constructive alternatives, as expressed in the design of alternative curricula, textbooks and methods.

CONCLUSION

The development of alternative education in South Africa should be seen as more than a reaction to the failure of state education. Alternative education cannot be regarded as merely the obverse of the education system that was central to apartheid ideology. According to Nkomo (1990), the reconstructed education system should possess knowledge of the assumptions, canons, philosophical orientations and practices of the old system in relation to the political economy, but only to ensure critical understanding of the new system, which will be antithetical to the old in its praxis. Democratic people's education "will replace the inferior, segregated, prejudicial, divisive and undemocratic apartheid education" (Nkomo, 1990, p. 299). The literature on postapartheid education abounds with similar rhetoric. While the anger and the passionate rejection of apartheid education is amply justified and understandable, the time has come to do more than formulate ringing phrases, especially if they are predominantly expressions of what should *not* be. It is now time to formulate constructive, positive and concrete alternatives, not only on the level of ideals and general principles, but in the form of specifics—implementable curricula.

Alternatives should not aim only at the transfer of power or control from one sector of society to another, but should provide the bases for a society committed to other values, other priorities and other concepts of what South African society can be (Gardiner, 1990a). Currently, there is a fair amount of resistance to revolutionary changes, even at times by the very people who stand to benefit most from them (Gwalla-Ogisi, 1990).

In the next chapter, some of the reasons for the resistance are touched on and suggestions for an education system moving toward a peaceful multicultural society are offered.

11

Education for Reconciliation

On March 17, 1992, the white electorate voted for political reform and the book on apartheid was proclaimed to be finally, and irrevocably, closed. President F. W. de Klerk exhorted all South Africans, even the 31 percent of whites who had voted against reform, to participate in the process of reconciliation (*Rapport*, March 22, 1992). The Inkatha Freedom party and Joe Latakgomo (*Sunday Star*, March 22, 1992) commented that the affirmative vote restored the faith of many black South Africans in their compatriots. Graeme Simpson, research officer of the Project for the Study of Violence at the University of the Witwatersrand, cautioned that forty years of divisive ideology do not disappear overnight.

WHY NOT KEEP THE SKELETONS IN THE CUPBOARD?

Among whites, there is a call to forget the past. The desire for a clean slate is understandable on the part of those who would prefer to forget their moral and financial responsibility for past actions, but resented by those who paid the cost of apartheid's successes in social and personal terms. Although guilt is counterproductive in antiracist work (Spoonley, 1988), attempting to keep the skeletons in the cupboard may fire the already wild imaginations of those Africanists who hold the white "settlers" collectively responsible for a history of colonialism and apartheid (James, 1992). On the part of whites, the level of political awareness and knowledge is low, although they are likely to manifest relative depth in terms of affective awareness (Gagiano, 1992). The danger of these attitudes is that they will contribute to freezing the population into two irreconcilable racial groups, locked in an ongoing struggle over resources and political power.

Moreover, the black-white political polarization of South African society should not obscure its complex, multiethnic and multicultural nature. Violence is by no means limited to white-black conflict. In the crime-ridden black townships and the strife-torn rural districts of Natal, the pattern of black-on-black violence shows a complex interplay between territorial and economic competition rooted in age-old local tribal feuds (Zulu versus Xhosa), exacerbated by overcrowding and unemployment, political power mongering (Inkatha Freedom party versus African National Congress), and promoted by state complicity in undercover activities (Goldstone Commission, 1992). The fact remains that the unification of many black people in their struggle against apartheid has tended to mask the complexity of the cultural and ethnic mosaic that is South Africa.

A CULTURAL KALEIDOSCOPE

Once the dust settles over the present dualistic black-white political battleground, the true plural nature of the new nation-state will probably reappear. Of the 40 million people living in South Africa, the mother tongue of 30 million is an African language, as opposed to the 10 million whose mother tongue is Afrikaans or English. More than 18 million blacks can speak Afrikaans, and almost 17 million English, but only 4 percent of whites, coloreds and Asians can speak an African language (Schuring, 1992). There are four large African language groups: Nguni, Sotho, Shangaan-Tsonga and Venda. In its turn, the Nguni languages comprise Ndebele, Swazi, Xhosa and Zulu. The Sotho group includes Northern Sotho (Pedi), Southern Sotho (Basutu), and Western Sotho (Tswana). There are also smaller groups such as the desert-dwelling Koisan, and second or third generation immigrant communities of various European extractions. These groups are ethnically and culturally related in varying degrees. Many people are bicultural or have dual and even multiple cultural identities, and speak several languages.

To complicate matters, the mosaic is in motion—a kaleidoscope of rapid and fundamental change on all levels, including economic, political, social and cultural. It contains a modern sector (most whites and a growing number of blacks) and a modernizing sector; a tribal, rural sector, and a rapidly growing, homogenizing urban sector. Acculturative pressures toward industrial, Western values will probably cause an accelerating flow from "traditional" to "modern." Apartheid structures that used to encapsulate different cultural groups, have crumbled. As the economic and cultural boycotts that have isolated the country from the global community are lifted, ideas, institutions, technologies, people, films, literature and other culture carriers are streaming in from every part of the world.

REDISTRIBUTION OF WEALTH AND RESOURCES

The harsh realities of South Africa's economic problems perhaps overshadow all else: rising inflation, a collapsing currency, a deep-seated profitability crisis in the manufacturing industry, acute foreign indebtedness and increasing rates of unemployment (Nasson, 1990). The frustration of the raised expectations and false hopes created by the prospects of rapid and fundamental change holds a danger in itself. Clearly, much of the escalating violence has been the product of pervasive fear and insecurity in a dramatically changing society. The Center for Educational Research and Innovation (CERI, 1989) emphasizes that if the harmonious coexistence of culturally and economically different groups is to be achieved, the distribution of wealth must not be too uneven. If social welfare is inadequate or ill adjusted, if the chances of making money remain limited, if the prospects for social advancement are slight, then the risk of conflict increases and ethnicity becomes overstressed. Also, as Nasson (1990) rightly says, the grotesque legacy of discriminatory schooling remains a living reality—manifested in the scale of black illiteracy, poorly qualified teachers and abysmal matriculation pass rates. Equal opportunity and equal access to education in South Africa require redistribution of resources, not only in education, implying substantial downward, no less than upward, shifts (Nasson & Samuel, 1990).

POSTAPARTHEID EDUCATION

The debate over education is nearly synonymous with the debate concerning the future of South Africa, which is increasingly seen as a unified, democratic, nonracial, nonsexist, nonexploitative and, possibly, socialist state (Nasson, 1990). But when Nkomo (1990) states that the school's mission must be "to become a forum for the critical discourse on the dynamic and dialectical relation between the state and the individual" (p. 303), it begins to sound like one questionable ideology being replaced by another. Marxist analyses of society and education have brought invaluable insights contributing to the overthrow of the apartheid system. The question is whether South Africa can afford to make the same mistakes that have led to the collapse of the Communist regimes in Europe and elsewhere in Africa. Revivalist and rhetorical approaches to the country's problems must be abandoned in favor of concrete and realistic strategies to accelerate much-needed processes of transformation (Alexander, 1990). One of the most urgent tasks to be tackled is eradication of the racism that has been the cornerstone of the school system and of the society at large.

ERADICATING RACISM

Apartheid education has largely failed to equip the South African youth with the skills and values required for the transformation to a democratic, multicultural society. Social and political intolerance and an incapacity to deal with conflict are fundamental obstructions (Goldstone Commission, 1992). The question has been asked whether or not political groups that organize along racial lines should be outlawed. Roskam (1992) argues that racism is not just another ideology, but rather a criminal concept. This idea should be handled with the utmost care.

Recent history in which the ruling party found it right and fitting to criminalize and ruthlessly weed out certain political organizations, remains a lesson that costs dearly in human life and suffering. Alternatively, the hope that the demise of statutory apartheid will automatically lead to the disappearance of racism is a vain one. Even in the United States, where democratic and antiracist policies have been in place for decades, incidents of murder and mayhem, including physical attacks, threats and racial epithets, prove that racism is alive, well and thriving (Sue & Sue, 1990). It is obvious that merely allowing different groups to associate freely is not the solution to the problem of prejudice.

THE CONTACT HYPOTHESIS

Identifying racism with a race of people makes antiracism an issue of either changing or overthrowing a race—a response to racism in racist terms. The opposite idea is that individuals are the source of negative attitudes, and that contact with the other race would provide people with the opportunity of discovering that they share basic values and attitudes. Unfortunately, contact itself does not guarantee favorable results. Some people are so rigid in their prejudices, that any out-group behavior is in fact interpreted as supporting their initial attitudes (Brislin, 1981). In a study by Luiz and Krige (Mynhardt & Du Toit, 1991) a special program based on ideal contact principles was employed in a multicultural school setting and produced significant mutual positive attitude change, which was found to be intact after a year's time. Contact situations have to comply with a number of preconditions for positive attitude change to occur (Mynhardt & Du Toit, 1991):

1. Equal status is necessary within the contact situation.
2. Shared coping for achieving common goals is needed.
3. The contact situation should provide sufficient opportunity for friendship formation.
4. Proximity and intimate contact are necessary.
5. Prevailing norms must be favorable.
6. Contact should occur voluntarily, under rewarding, pleasant conditions.
7. Success, and perceptions of possible success, are important.
8. Particularly in the case of schools, it is essential that the immediate authorities support the contact, that opportunity for meaningful contact is created and that the percentage of members of the group with whom integration occurs should not be too high (pp. 285–286).

DECATEGORIZATION AND PERSONALIZATION

Whereas personalization is the result of the ideal contact situation, interaction between members of different groups is often category-oriented, which predisposes people to react in terms of group identities. Category-identity responses result in a depersonalization of out-group members, and intergroup comparison and strategies to achieve more positive social identity, causing tension between groups. Category-based interactions must be replaced by interpersonal-based relations. This is not possible unless differentiation occurs and unique information concerning the individual members of the out-group is made available.

Attempts to reduce category-based behavior may be thwarted by individual characteristics like poor self-image. A poor self-image may render identification with a supposedly superior in-group impossible to a person. The same applies to uncertain or threatened status for other reasons, which may cause a need to maintain category separation. The effects of contact have been found to differ for low-status and high-status groups in South Africa, with lower-status (black) groups exhibiting a large degree of ethnocentrism (Mynhardt & Du Toit, 1991). To explain this phenomenon, the effect of relative deprivation in terms of personal and group access to financial, political and judicial justice must not be overlooked (Appelgryn, 1991).

TOWARD A PLURAL SOCIETY

A completely color-blind approach to the resolution of the intergroup conflicts in South Africa would thus appear to be unrealistic. A certain amount of social categorization may indeed be necessary to enable people to create a meaningful and positive social and cultural identity (Munro, 1989). Neither a "melting pot" nor a forced "pressure cooker" (Brislin, 1981) type of assimilation will work in South Africa. Experience in the rest of Africa, containing approximately 700 traditional societies integrated into fewer than fifty nations, suggests that any attempt to convince, for example, the Zulu tribe and the Afrikaans-speaking whites in South Africa to relinquish their identities in favor of some new, all-encompassing category, would probably fail. The ideal situation would be for all groups to be proud of their own identities, but myths regarding apparently irreconcilable differences should be exploded. The process of nation building should not destroy the subidentities of the rich variety of cultural groups. Pluralism is something to work toward, and a multicultural educational system may be an integrative mechanism for achieving a plural society in South Africa (Beckmann, 1991; Steyn & Viljoen, 1991).

AN INTERCULTURAL APPROACH

The outcomes of multicultural education elsewhere in the world have been somewhat disappointing. The aim of an intercultural approach is more ambitious than the objectives of multicultural approaches: to form a new, open cultural identity that is neither ethnocentric, nor passionately tied to its own beliefs and values (CERI, 1989). The ideal is that all children should be addressed by a multicultural curriculum in order that they may understand what it means to live in a multicultural and multiracial society. Multicultural education should not be based solely on ethical arguments (to fight discrimination due to racism or ethnocentrism) or legal arguments (respect for human rights), because South Africa can survive and thrive only if different cultures can coexist, and individuals, depending on circumstances and needs, can move from one culture to another. However, multicultural education might involve a number of potential inherent tensions or contradictions, and these must be faced in an educational system where more mistakes can hardly be afforded (Samuel, 1990). The following section will elaborate on these tensions and suggest possible solutions or compromises. The solutions are to be found somewhere along the continuum between the extremes of particularism versus universalism; collectivism versus individualism; indigenous versus school culture; traditionalism versus modernization; and traditional versus school education.

PARTICULARISM VERSUS UNIVERSALISM

Verne (CERI, 1989) drew attention to the apparently contradictory nature of the development of contemporary culture: on the one hand, there is the search for cultural authenticity, the return to origins, and maintenance of traditions; on the other hand, we find the spread of a uniform world culture, the emergence of supranational myths and the adoption of similar lifestyles in widely differing settings. Modern technological societies have generated a transnational, composite, mass culture with its own language whose linguistic imprint is already universally evident (Hutmacher, 1987). Multicultural education must reflect a balance between local, regional and national cultures and the confrontation of those with the exploding world culture.

COLLECTIVISM VERSUS INDIVIDUALISM

For a long time educational policies in Western countries aimed at uniformity. The idea was to treat everyone in the same way, have everyone learn the same language, offer them the same services, instill the same values and impart the same knowledge. This strategy was inspired by a concern for justice and equality and to consolidate national unity. The collective identity is now considered to be at least as important as the individual one (Kagitcibasi, 1989; Kashima, 1989). One of its functions is to help in the rediscovery of the culture of origin, to maintain and strengthen the feeling of belonging to a community (De Certeau, 1987). However, there is a danger of becoming locked into a kind of ethnic, or socialist-collectivist (Carnoy, 1990; Samoff, 1990) fatality by asserting the primacy of the community over the individual. The aim should be the harmonious development of the personality and intellectual differences of all children in a climate of liberty, which enables the maximum benefit to be drawn from the cultural environment while at the same time keeping it at a certain distance (CERI, 1989).

INDIGENOUS VERSUS SCHOOL CULTURE

The idea that multicultural education is primarily effective is an oversimplification (Jeffcoate, 1981). The interaction between the culture of a people and its practices in acquiring and transmitting knowledge is very strong. The concept of knowledge itself differs from one culture to another—compare, for example, the Western, the Moslem and the traditional Japanese concepts of knowledge (Kaufman et al., 1989; Segall et al., 1990). Thus each culture influences, in its own way, the formation of cognitive abilities and even generates its own teaching model. If we want to recreate a culture of learning, we will have to find a synthesis between the traditional Western cultural epistemology and the indigenous ones that were ignored and disempowered when a Western, white, school culture was imposed. Multicultural education at its best gives access to other forms of knowledge and to other cultural traditions having knowledge different in content and internal structure from that of the school tradition (Hemmings, 1984; Taylor, 1991). In many ways, these ideas coincide with the ideals of People's Education (Alexander, 1990; Gardiner, 1990a; 1990b).

TRADITIONALISM VERSUS MODERNIZATION

In most so-called developing nations, the reality of whether a child enters school and how far he progresses, virtually determines which of two contrasting lifestyles—traditional or modern—will be pursued during adulthood and is one reason why generational gaps are so dramatic in developing societies. Students may feel that it is nearly impossible to communicate with their uneducated parents. In such settings, school vacations are in many respects like a trip to a foreign land (Segall et al., 1991). Ironically, modernization may not be a one-way road to salvation. Consider the myth of technology associated with modernization (Fuglesang, 1982). Is it really for the good of humankind? Is it desirable, clean, apolitical, efficient or even necessary? The myth of development is intertwined with technology (Chombart De Lauwe, 1987). Both are seen as synonymous with economic growth, a linear process of social change ending in the model of the modern Western consumer society. However, this orientation is no longer feasible, given dwindling global resources. Likewise, education has been promulgated as the key to development, and, over the last two decades, has led to an enormous growth in allocations for schooling in Third World countries. Yet the idea that a correlation exists between the stock of educated manpower and the rate of economic growth remains another myth (Hyslop, 1990), because, by and large, the unemployed are the educated. In formulating educational goals, a balance must be found between preservation of traditional African values and lifestyles on the one hand, and development on the other. To save the world, industrial civilization must be transformed into a postindustrial society that no longer emphasizes growth and material welfare per se. We must turn to preindustrial societies for guidance (Heilbroner, in Segall et al., 1990).

TRADITIONAL VERSUS SCHOOL EDUCATION

Informal education, characteristic of the Third World, is sometimes called "precolonial education," even though it still occurs (Keto, 1990). Some prefer to call it "traditional education." Its main characteristics, in comparison with formal education, are summarized by Segall et al. (1991, pp. 126–128) as follows:

Traditional Education	*Traditional School Education*
1. Provided everywhere	Occurs in a specialized place
2. Provided all the time	Occurs at a specialized time
3. Provided by everyone	Provided by specialized personnel
4. Tied closely to environment	Cut off from real world
5. Integration with productive work	Separate from production
6. Insists on cooperative community spirit	Emphasizes individual competition
7. Language of the people is spoken	A foreign tongue is spoken
8. Knowledge is transmitted orally	Learning involves written activities
9. Learner responsible for obtaining knowledge	Teacher responsible for imparting knowledge
10. Spiritual values important	Primacy of scientific ethos

Wagner (in Segall et al., 1990) speaks of "appropriate education" (by analogy to "appropriate technology"), to suggest that traditional education has a definite contribution to make, given the needs of Third World countries. For example, Brenner (in Segall et al., 1990), in a study of arithmetic in Liberian schools, demonstrated the value of a combination of traditional strategies and school-based algorithms. Also, positive self-concept can best be nurtured in an environment that respectfully accepts a child's first culture (Seelye, 1988). Teaching methods and style, classroom organization and the nature and the quality of the school's relationship with parents and the community are aspects of the "hidden curriculum" that transmits vital messages in this regard (Nixon, 1985; Taylor, 1991).

EVOLVING A CORE CULTURE

Provided that the necessary balance between the potentially harmful extremes mentioned in the previous section can be achieved, multicultural educational strategies may be implemented to establish a common core culture that can unite the different cultural and social groups. The foundation for a common or core South African culture can be laid in the preschool phase. It is suggested that all children in South Africa, regardless of language group, learn a common core of stories, songs, myths, fables and nursery rhymes, drawn from the three main cultural traditions or currents that constitute the country—the traditions of Africa, Europe and Asia (Alexander, 1990). The basic material of this core treasury will be internalized by all children, but through different language media, much as the thousands of Christian communities throughout the world imbibe the material of the Bible. The danger of multicultural education as a common core curriculum, is that it may fail to relate the issues with which it deals to the curriculum as a whole. Accordingly, a strategy of "permeation" is recommended (Mukhopadhyay, 1984; Nixon, 1985). The common culture would rest on a number of basic values or premises permeating the entire curriculum, to be briefly discussed in the final section of this chapter, for example, democracy; equality and human rights; multilingualism; a shared history; religious tolerance; and global citizenship. If these values can be instilled in the next generation, the wounds of a disrupted and traumatized society may be gradually healed.

DEMOCRACY

Alexander (1990) rightly points out that many in South Africa believe in basic democratic values. Yet equality, liberty and participatory democracy are still under constant threat in a society torn by strife and violence. These values need to be taught, nurtured and promoted in every possible way. One of the problems that needs to be addressed is the interpretation of the different connotations associated with the word "democracy." Whites associate it largely with tolerance, while black South Africans emphasize its emphasis on the structural inequalities in society (Schmidt, 1992). Much may be learned from the notion of consultation, a principle at the heart of People's Education (Gardiner, 1990b).

EQUALITY AND HUMAN RIGHTS

The notion that sexism will be eradicated along with racism in a new educational dispensation is a popular one. However, the interaction between gender and race is not simple. African women tend not to challenge marriage or the family, focusing more on the need for land reforms, rural development and the relations between women in polygamous marriages (Knowles & Mercer, 1990). In South Africa, black women have been affected by the double oppression of racism and sexism. Moreover, feminism is capable of racism, just as antiracism is capable of sexism. Children should be educated to abhor inequality in whichever form it presents itself. Human rights are an obligatory reference point for multicultural education (Bray, 1992). The best guarantee against the excesses of cultural relativism ought to be human rights, respect for which constitutes an inviolable limit for any open cultural policy (CERI, 1989; Zec, 1981).

MULTILINGUALISM

The fierce defense of languages becomes meaningful if we do not disguise the fact that the real issue is not only linguistic but also political, as well as economic (Paulston, 1987; CERI, 1989). In South Africa, language has been used as a tool to arouse emotion (Pieterse, 1992). However, in a study by Louw-Potgieter and Louw (reported in Louw-Potgieter, 1991), it was found that students preferred a language policy of diversity. Complete dominance of a single language, even the internationally acceptable English option, emerged as an unpopular choice. Neville Alexander's two basic principles (Louw-Potgieter, 1991) concerning language planning bear repetition:

1. All languages spoken by the people of South Africa have an equal right to exist.
2. The main aim of language policy for South Africa should be to facilitate communication between groups of people who have been separated for so long by apartheid policies.

An education system that is unable to make the best use of children's linguistic knowledge, fails to encourage languages spoken at home, and does not favor the survival of the country's minority languages, is less than effective from any point of view (CERI, 1989).

A SHARED HISTORY

The emphasis on Afrikaner identity in traditional cultural activities, and especially in the teaching of history in school, has resulted in category-oriented behavior (Mynhardt & Du Toit, 1991). Through mass mobilization, teacher, student and parent organizations have already influenced the curricula and the syllabi being implemented in black schools, especially in subjects such as English and history. Examples of more appropriate textbooks and other resources are provided by Alexander (1990). There is a danger that "people's history," if it means exclusive emphasis on the history of the struggle for freedom in South Africa within a Marxist-socialist frame of reference, may replace one kind of political illiteracy and intolerance with another. There is an urgent need for a history curriculum emphasizing the heritage of a shared past in which both the "villains" and the "victims" are seen and understood within their sociocultural and historical contexts. The achievements and the strengths, as well as the problems and tragedies, of different groups must be featured as honestly as possible (Worrall, 1981). Children should acquire an adequate understanding of South Africa's position in Africa and in the contemporary world system.

RELIGIOUS TOLERANCE

The South African state religion, until the present time, has been Christianity, and more particularly, Calvinism. However, South Africa is a multifaith society, including not only the major international creeds—Hinduism, Islam, Judaism, Christianity and Buddhism—but also the convictions of those who worship their ancestors, adhere to witchcraft, and the persuasions of those who give a religious dimension to their explicitly racist beliefs. Nevertheless, most religions espouse the ideals of neighborly love, moral upliftment, reciprocity of social behavior and charity to the weak and humble. Building on these ideals, religious instruction within a framework of respect and tolerance can play an important role in the formation of a minimum framework of common values (Halstead, 1988; Heyns, 1992). Religious education and religious instruction should, however, be clearly distinguished from one another (Wood, 1984). The confessional approach is concerned with the instruction of a particular creed, whereas a more phenomenological approach is intended to inform rather than to convert (Jansen, 1990).

GLOBAL CITIZENSHIP

Resource depletion, environmental degradation, and the need for more equitable economic development can be confronted effectively only if viewed as worldwide challenges. Yet outmoded consciousness persists, fueling a loyalty to ethnic or national segments. Especially in South Africa, the world has been divided into "us" and "them." Through world studies and education for peace (Hicks, 1984) schools must help children to develop the empathy to identify with the whole human race as enthusiastically as they do with their own tribes. Global citizenship requires a "quantum leap in good will" (Segall et al., 1990), accompanied by enlightened leadership and social policy that provide the requisite economic and normative settings in which such good will can flourish.

CONCLUSION

Our approach to educational renewal in South Africa must urgently move beyond rhetoric. We have to adopt a transitional and transformational approach that recognizes the complexity of the historical process in southern Africa as a whole (Alexander, 1990). At the same time, it must be recognized that South Africa is not unique. Almost all teaching systems function in societies that are, in fact, culturally complex, hybrid, heterogeneous and pluralist (CERI, 1989). The strains and contrasts, conflicts and syntheses generated by cultural and ethnic encounters are essential for the vitality of democracy, and fruitful for the cultural enrichment of the societies that accept them. An intercultural approach rests on the conviction that dialogue between cultures is, in principle, correct from a political, moral and educational perspective. The present represents an open, defining moment, a time to move beyond recrimination toward hope and understanding.

12

Culturally Effective Skills for Guidance Teachers and Other Helping Professionals

The concept of comprehensive multicultural training for counselors, psychologists, social workers, guidance personnel and other helping professionals has been addressed extensively in the literature. Guidance teachers in South Africa provide occupational, personal and social information to pupils through regularly scheduled group guidance classes and participation in case conferences. Such personnel can provide supportive, consultative, referral and service activities. In the supportive role, the guidance teacher can work in partnership with other specialists in the school. In the consultative role, guidance personnel participate in case conferences on individual children and modify instruction to meet the individual needs of the child. The guidance instructor can also act as a referral agent to those experts in the community who can help the child with special needs. Last, the guidance person can provide individual and group counseling to those in need.

Cultural factors shape behavior and provide a basis for interactions that are likely to occur in the counseling relationship. In a previous section the worldviews of Africans, Indians, coloreds and Afrikaners have been described. Although individual differences and the universal factors of being human cannot be ignored, differing cultural backgrounds have also led to various cultural assumptions and values. For example, in comparison with Western approaches, Africans have tended to approach activity with spontaneous expression and a rhythmic, noncompulsive pace of life. Time is not measured literally, but experientially. Group goals, social relatedness and cooperative effort are valued. The African sees himself/herself as part of nature in an unbroken chain of life and believes that man should accept the natural order. Spiritual values are woven into the fabric of daily life and creativity is a strong characteristic of African society.

Hinduism values a state of being or consciousness, with spiritual goals seen as the important goals in life. Theirs is a mystically oriented society. The person is located within a social system and his or her identity is found in roles, groups, family and society. Hierarchical relationships are stressed, and the basis of values is authoritative and found in the sacred religious texts and writings. Social control is exercised through societal ostracism, guilt and shame. Hinduism is both a religion, a philosophy and a social system. It represents a life-centered philosophical-religious-ethical approach. In their upbringing, Indians are exposed to an emphasis on ethical behavior, transcendental values and rejection of an egoistic approach to life with its wants and rewards.

Issues for the Afrikaner are complex. Infused in the identity is the authoritarian ideology of Afrikaner nationalism and the intergenerational transmission of white domination. In a rapidly changing society, feelings of guilt, shame and confusion may be presenting concerns. Fear about one's role in the new South African may add to a host of self-doubts. Rigid sex roles represent dichotomous thinking and a polarized way of being. For many Afrikaner clients, early ethnocentric conditioning has resulted in anxiety and fearfulness, feelings of alienation and a distorted racial-cultural identity development. Fear about the future is a dominant concern.

In the shaping of colored identity, skin tone may be seen as having implications for self-image and peer acceptance. In a rigidly polarized black-white South African society, there may be ambiguous identity feelings. Counseling approaches should be cognizant of the intrapsychic representation of experiences and its possible impact on behavior, and should be approached with caution as there may be many colored individuals who want to be identified as South Africans and not as "coloreds." Because they have been placed in a marginal situation, there may be feelings of isolation and of not quite belonging. The strains of living in two different cultural milieus—African and Afrikaner—may lead to confusion about social identity and to role confusion. Mental health issues may include ambivalence and heightened self-consciousness, with these feelings expressed in either withdrawal or aggression.

With respect to Indian, colored, African and Afrikaner culture, nonverbal signs and symbols should also be noted, for the spatial distance between two people during conversation is an important cultural indicator. Anglo-American and British culture require greater distance (about arm's length) between speakers, while Africans, coloreds and Indians may express preferences for very small distance. The degree and intensity of eye contact expected during conversation is also culturally conditioned. Anglo-Americans expect direct eye contact in face-to-face conversation, but staring is considered rude. Instead, the speaker and listener are expected to break eye contact occasionally. If no eye contact is maintained, there is often a suspicion that an individual is not being forthright or honest. Yet, among Indians and Africans, direct eye contact may be seen as aggressive and disrespectful or impolite. Therefore, a guidance teacher's admonition to the Indian or African child to look her/him in the eye may create conflict for the child, for if the child is being reprimanded, direct eye contact would be disrespectful.

Culture conditions a people's response to direct body contact, such as touching, holding and patting on the head. Although Africans view frequent touching as an important aspect of communication, Indian women may be embarrassed by public physical contact. Communication may also be difficult to maintain if one person is from a "contact" society and the other from a "noncontact" one. Multiethnic guidance is the recognition and the inclusion of the heritage, traditions and customs, language or linguistic style, and the ongoing lifestyle of the many cultures and ethnic groups that constitute South African society. More than one cultural perspective should be provided in guidance activities and practices. Activities can be included that address the processes of perceptions of human differences and commonalities and how these influence the way pupils deal with people.

A cross-cultural or multicultural approach is a transcendent approach. It recognizes that people everywhere have the same universal needs, such as the need to love and be loved and the need to feel worthwhile. However, such an approach also recognizes that particular groups have special needs that must be understood and addressed by the helping professional. As such, the counseling of persons of culturally diverse backgrounds by people who are not trained or competent to work with such groups should be regarded as unethical. Such well-intentioned helping efforts run the risk of resulting in cultural oppression, for example, the helper trying to superimpose constraints and values that may be in direct opposition to the cultural values of the helpee.

A cross-cultural approach is not cultural stereotyping, but rather, cultural sensitivity. A cross-culturally skilled counselor recognizes that each cultural group may have particular ways of behaving, but also recognizes the necessity of recognizing the uniqueness of each human being within a cultural framework. People should not be stereotyped just because they come from a certain culture, but rather, knowledge of culture should be used as a guideline or map in order to adapt counseling techniques. In truth, the guidance counselor may find that a person from a particular culture really behaves more in a Western manner than in a traditional or culturally indigenous manner.

Effective helping relationships are tied to an understanding of our own world-view, as well as an understanding of our client's world-view. World-view is the way in which people perceive their relationship to nature, institutions, other people and things. It constitutes an individual's psychological orientation in life and can determine how he or she thinks, behaves, makes decisions and defines events. World-view is a function of an individual's cultural upbringing. One source of conflict in cross-cultural communication is that individuals often perceive things differently as a result of having different world-views. The skilled cross-cultural counselor thus is sensitive to his or her own world-view as well as to the world-view of the client, and exercises culturally aware knowledge and skills in order to reduce the barriers to effective helping. Culturally effective counseling requires that practitioners develop a culturally pluralistic philosophy and an appreciation of cultural variations.

Guidance teachers, social workers, psychologists and related helping personnel need to be cognizant of the following barriers operating in the counseling situation, with respect to culturally diverse clients, that could impede the helping process:

1. Incongruent expectations about counseling—the counselor expects clients to adopt counselor values that often do not reflect client cultural value systems
2. Overemphasis on verbal self-disclosure—culturally different clients may not want to disclose intimate details about their lives, and the counselor then labels them defensive and resistant
3. Overemphasis on abstract and nonproblem-solving strategies—counselor behaves in an ambiguous and nondirective manner
4. Monolingual orientation—counselor maintains only one language
5. Overemphasis on long-range goals and the future
6. Lack of understanding of the whole person—counselor makes a distinction between physical, mental and spiritual as if they were separate entities
7. Lack of understanding of social forces and ignorance of importance of social context of environment in understanding problems of living
8. Lack of appreciation for nonverbal communication—counselor does not understand the importance of the nonverbal
9. Ethnocentric world-view—counselor lacks awareness of his or her own cultural heritage
10. Ignorance of self, racism and other's cultural identity

Ethnic customs and rituals can be included in the guidance curriculum. What do the dance, the artwork and the special food mean in the context of the culture and traditions, the heritage and the daily life of the group from which it comes? How does a particular custom compare and contrast to what is commonly accepted in South African life? The theme of all multiethnic guidance activities should be that of diverse cultures and subgroups living together with mutual respect and understanding. Ethnic guidance education should help to develop an acceptance and appreciation for the rich cultural diversity in South Africa. The process and successful outcome of counseling is significantly increased as a result of cross-cultural effectiveness. The process of increasing a counselor's sensitivity to cultural issues may be divided into three areas: awareness, knowledge and skills.

ACQUIRING CULTURAL AWARENESS, KNOWLEDGE AND SKILLS

Awareness means examining the beliefs and attitudes of one's own culture and those of other ethnic groups. It suggests being aware of personal prejudices and biases and moving toward the goal of valuing and respecting differences. Knowledge refers to the acquisition of information regarding one's own and other cultural values, world-view and social norms. Being knowledgeable about the history, experiences, culture, values and lifestyle of various racial-ethnic groups is very important. Skills refer to the ability to send and receive both verbal and nonverbal messages accurately and appropriately.

The following framework may serve as a useful guide in acquiring cross-cultural awareness, knowledge and skills.

Awareness

In the helping encounter, helping practitioners must have an awareness of who they are and of their own values and predispositions. Culturally effective communication requires that personal world-views, cultural contexts and biases be recognized, assessed and accepted. As an initial starting point, it is vitally important that practitioners be in touch with their own cultural baggage and prejudices. An examination of how factors in their own lives have impinged on their professional philosophy, as well as how these factors have been translated into actual practices with their clients, should be acknowledged. An awareness of personal limitations and biases when working with ethnic persons should be acknowledged and such an awareness should be part of an ongoing appraisal for practitioners, with referral occurring when necessary. Ideally, when interacting with culturally diverse clients, guidance and counseling personnel in a multiracial school setting would thus apply a culturally pluralistic philosophy and refrain not only from the imposition of culturally dominant beliefs, but from attitudes of paternalism and condescension as well. In sum, in acquiring cultural awareness it is important that helping personnel in an agency, private practice or a multiethnic school setting examine how their own cultures have shaped them, both personally and professionally, and that they recognize how such conditioning may affect the way they perceive their clients. Practitioners who disregard cultural variables and impose their own world-view reflect cultural encapsulation, whereas culturally effective counselors are aware of their own identity yet able to share the world-view of their clients without negating its legitimacy.

Knowledge

Cross-cultural literature also suggests that cultural knowledge is an essential ingredient of cross-cultural effectiveness. If helping professionals are to broaden their understanding of divergent world-views, they must first gain relevant knowledge and information about the specific population groups for whom their services are designed. The following categories are suggested by Parker, Valley and Geary (1986) as a base of knowledge essential for helping personnel with respect to diverse ethnic groups:

1. Racial pride and identity: Who are the key ethnic heroes and what are the important historical events?
2. Socioeconomic: What are the facts about income, population, occupation and level of education?
3. Communication: Are there language differences, nonverbal behaviors and special ethnic phrases important to different ethnic groups?
4. Cultural values: What are the unique characteristics of each ethnic group?
5. Sexual, marital and family issues: How do customs and morals differ from those of the dominant culture-defining group?
6. Contemporary issues and concerns: What are present and emerging areas of emphasis?

Information about various ethnic groups can be drawn from a wide range of sources, including social science textbooks, ethnic literature, popular magazines and print media, television and personal sources. Guided self-study literature, audiovisual presentations and interviews with experts can be helpful as well.

A useful framework for the assessment of the large-scale environment has been proposed by Triandis (1980) and can also enhance understanding of the culturally different client. It includes the following variables:

1. The ecology: awareness of the physical environment, resources, geography
2. The subsistence system: methods of exploitation of the economy to survive (i.e., agricultural, fishing, gathering, industrial work)
3. The sociocultural system: institutions, norms, roles, and values as they exist outside the individual
4. The individual system: perception, learning, motivation, subjective culture
5. The interindividual system: patterns of social behavior, including child-rearing methods
6. Protective systems: systems embodied by myths, folklore, etc.
7. Interaction patterns: patterns occurring between the individual and the environment

Since cross-cultural knowledge includes knowledge of individuals in their wider context—cultural, social and political—Triandis' model provides a fruitful avenue of exploration.

Once the helping practitioner has gained a cognitive understanding of cultural groups, an understanding of the client's experience or phenomenological world becomes the most important source of information. How the individual who is seeking help specifically represents the world must be understood. For example, although individuals of particular ethnic groups may have convergent world-views in certain respects, world-view is also mediated by such tools as gender, age, education and socioeconomic levels. Consequently, in addition to ethnic factors, how the client personally represents the world—his or her own individual world-view—must be understood before intervention is taken by the helper to produce change. For the practitioner, the three factors of cultural awareness, knowledge of the client's general cultural system, and special client world-view, must be considered. Such factors are critically important determinants of counseling process and outcome.

Skills

Guidance and counseling personnel, as well as social workers and psychologists, must not only be sensitized to racial and ethnic perspectives but also must be aware of approaches that are culturally encapsulated and ethnocentrically biased. Value and attitude differences between cultures must be acknowledged and understood, although with cautionary emphasis. Cultural differences must not be accentuated to such a degree that stereotyping becomes the negative consequence. Instead, culture-specific techniques, focussing on the humanistic and universal aspects of each individual, must instead be employed and must translate into an improved quality of service delivery.

Although knowledge of a client's culture does not in itself produce counselor effectiveness, counselors in multiracial settings must also be open and flexible enough to change their approach in order to meet the needs of the diverse clients they serve. This may require therapeutic personnel to develop and utilize nonconventional assessment skills. The available tools and techniques in the work setting may not be appropriate for clients from a different culture. Multimethod approaches instead may be needed to assess the capabilities, potentials and limitations of the ethnic client.

Four barriers that may be experienced in cross-cultural counseling have been identified by Tucker, Chennault and Mulkerne (1981) and these researchers describe effective strategies for overcoming them as well:

1. Negative attitude toward seeking counseling. *Strategy:* Emphatically acknowledge the client's fears and channel his/her thoughts toward action problem solving.
2. Defensiveness and fear of self-disclosure. *Strategy:* Be aware of and openly acknowledge counselor-client sociocultural differences and resulting problems.
3. Expectations of therapeutic failure. *Strategy:* Maximize the client's involvement and self-esteem.
4. Feelings of discomfort during therapy. *Strategy:* Relax the client by addressing his/her discomfort and by self-disclosing feelings about working with him or her.

Probably there is no situation in counseling that evidences as clear-cut a need for an accepting and nonjudgmental attitude than the interaction between a counselor and a client of different races, different cultures and different socioeconomic levels. In examining ways in which the counselor can become more effective with the culturally different client, Belkin (1981) points out that such clients:

1. Need to feel that they are perceived as individuals, rather than only as members of a group

2. Want to be able to retain their own identity, as well as to function within the context of the larger society
3. May tend to perceive the white counselor as being white, above all other perceptions, implying that any general, stereotypical feelings about whites will be projected onto the counselor
4. Need a sense of social mobility; they want to be able to feel that they have an opportunity to rise above their present station in life. Often this hope has been tempered by the realization of the severe restraints that poverty imposes upon social advancement
5. Want the emotional freedom to be able to express prejudices toward white people. They want to be able to feel that the white counselor will not be overly threatened by this expression
6. Want the school—through its curriculum, its teachers and its rules—to relate to their world rather than to the world of whites
7. See things happening around them over which they feel no control. They want to be better able to control their world, and their own destiny, but they are lacking many of the educational and psychological tools necessary for doing so
8. Often have less opportunity than their white counterparts to discuss home and family problems. Loyalty to the family may deter them from discussing these with an outsider
9. May see school as the primary social institution (which is considered oppressive and nonresponsive) and be inclined to act out their rage and anger within the school environment. (Pp. 455–457)

An understanding of these nine special attitudes and feelings will enable therapeutic practitioners to have a better understanding and interactional encounter with the culturally diverse client. Additionally, role playing, behavioral rehearsal, communication training, watching cross-cultural interactions and viewing relevant videotapes will be helpful as well.

APPLYING THE CROSS-CULTURAL MODEL IN A SCHOOL SETTING

Pedersen's (1988b) Triad Model enumerates four skill areas: (1) articulating the problem from the client's cultural perspective, (2) recognizing resistance from a culturally different client in specific rather than general terms, (3) diminishing counselor defensiveness and (4) learning recovery skills for getting out of trouble when making mistakes in counseling culturally different clients. Pedersen recommends the development of specific abilities within this framework in a model that has been influenced by Ivey's microcounseling skills approach (Ivey, 1980).

Tidwell (1980) also recommends the following guidelines in the provision of guidance and counseling services in the multiethnic school setting:

1. Counseling and guidance programs should be highly individualized.
2. Estimates of ability and behavior must come from assessment instruments that have minimal socioeconomic, class or cultural bias.

3. Counselors should recognize and value different learning styles, vocational goals and life purposes of counselees.
4. The processes by which students learn social behaviors should emphasize and value diverse cultural definitions of these behaviors.
5. While insisting on behavior that is neither anti-social nor hostile to other groups, the counselor must be tolerant and knowledgeable concerning behavioral differences.
6. The counselor should not devalue the culture or racial heritage of students, staff members or community.
7. Counseling and guidance methods that are appropriate for students from one culture may be less appropriate for students from another culture, so the counselor must help the school staff to increase its sensitivities to the appropriateness of varying methods.
8. Counseling methodologies should place high priority on building a sense of personal worth in students so they feel valued both as individuals and as members of particular cultural and racial groups.

Educational institutions must learn to find strength in racial and cultural pluralism. Counselors and guidance personnel can provide enriching experiences for multiculturalism that will recognize and enhance diverse cultural expressions. Pupils of differing races and cultures can be provided a meaningful learning encounter, thereby gaining a significant multicultural, multiracial education. Guidance and counseling professionals who practice in a multicultural school setting can serve as agents of change to reshape the educational system. As Washington and Lee (1981) note:

> Schools can incorporate the strengths and cultural influences that all students bring to the institution; this will foster development for every student. In this way education becomes a broader, humanizing phenomenon. As a humanizing force, therefore, the system should foster, rather than attempt to alter, diverse perspectives of reality. (P. 66)

It is imperative that helping practitioners in a multiethnic school setting learn about the culture and values of prospective clients. Practitioners must take full cognizance of their own values and be aware of their client's values. Understanding of clients' world-view enhances ethical and effective cross-cultural counseling since counselors would be aware of imposing (1) culturally dominant beliefs, (2) paternalism, (3) condescension, (4) misunderstanding and (5) mislabeling of cross-cultural clients as "sick." Guidance and counseling personnel's knowledge, awareness and skills are interrelated, and gaining knowledge of cultures may increase their awareness, which in turn can guide toward appropriate applications of alternative helping skills.

To be effective, guidance personnel thus must be equipped with a sense of their own personal identity, self-awareness and positive acceptance of their own group affiliation. This means that the guidance teacher must be aware of how he or she was socialized as a child and young adult, what values and customs were internalized and continued to be followed as a result of personal and group affiliations.

Guidance personnel need to first accept and feel comfortable with their own ethnicity and then respond positively to individuals who belong to other ethnic groups.

The darker side of the hurtful aspects of prejudice and discrimination generated by apartheid society must be addressed. Racism can be manifested in both personal and institutional dimensions. Meaningful discussions can center around the concept of ethnocentricism, the attitude that one's traditions, customs, language and values are the only way of doing things and that all other ways are inadequate or wrong. Discussion can also explore the nature of prejudice and racism and actions that have been taken in the past by the South African government to justify the oppression of the majority population and to deny them lack of opportunity and economic mobility.

The guidance curriculum can then provide activities for children around the following themes:

1. Knowing one's own identity, one's heritage and traditions. Who are your people? What are their practices, customs and ways?
2. Knowing about other groups in South Africa—what groups other than your own are present in South African society?
3. Knowing about the relationships between these ethnic groups. Are the relationships between various groups cooperative and supportive, or are they antagonistic and hostile? Have these relationships extended historically over centuries, over decades or are they very current?

The schools can make an important contribution in helping the individual identify and value his or her family heritage. In her book *The Schools and Socialization,* Audrey James Schwartz puts it this way:

> Schools are in an ideal position to redress many of the injustices that have historically been thrust upon the racially and ethnically different. Through an emphasis on cultural pluralism, they can foster a child's favorite identification with his or her own family and culture. They can reduce racial-ethnic self-hatred, increase self-esteem; and they create greater tolerance for cultural diversity. (Schwartz, 1985)

Guidance activities can also help the individual become aware of diverse groups living within South Africa, since it is likely that at some time he or she will come into contact with members of these groups. When working with students of culturally diverse backgrounds the guidance teacher can use the following strategies:

1. Learn each child's name, first and last, using the pronunciation the child's family would use.
2. Learn some phrases, sayings and expressions in languages that are spoken by children in his/her school. Using these phrases will increase your rapport.

3. Holidays and festivals that are unique to the ethnic group can be used as opportunities to explore diverse culture.
4. Notes and announcements should be sent home to parents who speak languages other than English in their own language.
5. Music and art activities representing a variety of cultures and ethnic groups can be used in guidance activities.
6. Parents can be used as consultants, volunteer assistants and sources of expertise.
7. Organized field trips to locations and activities associated with different cultures can be conducted.

Guidance activities to enhance multiethnic awareness and appreciation can include discussion, writing short stories, drawing pictures, making a mural, collages, dramatizations and putting on student programs. Discussions can center on contrast and comparisons of ways of acting, customs, traditions, languages, food and clothing. In an open forum, children can learn and grow in a nonjudgmental climate. Multicultural education will serve ultimately to combat intolerance, bigotry, prejudice and racism.

CONCLUSION

In order to become culturally skilled as a helping professional, one must become more fully aware of his or her own heritage as well as aware of possible biases that may interfere with effectiveness. Gaining knowledge about the history and culture of diverse groups in South Africa is also important in the development of new counseling skills. Special competencies are needed, such as, the ability to relate to culturally diverse clients in both individual and group counseling sessions, the ability to use a variety of multicultural counseling techniques rather than just those that represent a white, Western perspective, the skills to use career development programs that meet the needs of the culturally diverse individual, the ability to administer and interpret tests without allowing cultural bias to enter into the assessment process and the ability to use a wide range of consultation models appropriate to culturally diverse individuals and groups. Intervention strategies that are effective with specific client populations from cultural groups must be used, as well as indigenous helping sources.

A culturally skilled counselor will have the following beliefs and attitudes:

1. The culturally skilled helper is one who has moved from being culturally unaware to being aware and sensitive to his/her own cultural heritage and to valuing and respecting differences.
2. The culturally skilled counselor is aware of his/her own values and biases and how they may affect clients.
3. Culturally skilled counselors are comfortable with differences that exist between themselves and their clients in terms of race and beliefs.

4. The culturally skilled counselor is sensitive to circumstances (personal biases, stage of ethnic identity, sociopolitical influences, etc.) that may dictate referral in general.
5. The culturally skilled counselor acknowledges and is aware of his/her own racist attitudes, beliefs and feelings.

The culturally skilled professional also will understand the world-view of the client he or she is working with and will possess knowledge and information about the client's particular cultural group. At the skills level, the practitioner must have a wide variety of verbal and nonverbal responses and must be able to send and receive verbal and nonverbal messages accurately and appropriately. There must be an awareness of the impact of helping interventions on the client and the adaptability of helping models that can be more effective with respect to the client's cultural background.

13

Options and Directions for Psychology within a Framework for Mental Health Services in South Africa

CURRENT SERVICES

Mental health services are provided through health and welfare structures, in the education sector, in industry, correctional institutions, the armed forces, through religious organizations and by other, less formal, mental health workers. In white, affluent, urban areas, curative services are available, accessible and manifestly affordable—2,420 psychologists are in private practice in these areas. Services in the public sector are lamentably inadequate—especially for the black population. What does exist is almost exclusively aimed at custodial care for the mentally ill and the mentally retarded (Freeman, 1992). Even when state-subsidized programs such as those by the National Council for Mental Health and other welfare organizations are included in the picture, according to the Psychological Association of South Africa (PASA, 1989) the services for the majority are grossly inadequate.

HUMAN RESOURCES FOR MENTAL HEALTH CARE

According to Freeman (1992), the following figures are probably overestimates, as they indicate registered persons rather than actual providers:

Psychiatrists	290	1:130,500 population
Psychologists	2,420	1:15,200 population
(Clinical)	1,060	1:35,800 population
Psychiatric nurses	7,000	1:5,400 population
Social workers	7,300	1:5,200 population

About 20 percent of the population can afford private care, while 80 percent are dependent on the public and welfare sector. However, only 10 percent of registered clinical psychologists are employed in hospital or state posts for the mentioned 80 percent of the population. The ideal of a collaborative team model is not attainable due to the drastic shortage of psychologists in general hospitals (Pillay, 1987). In the public sector there is approximately one psychologist per 304,000 of the population. First World ratios are in the region of 1 psychologist per 4,000. Of the 1,060 registered clinical psychologists, about 200 live in the greater Johannesburg area—a practitioner to population ratio of roughly 1:3,000. This may go a long way toward explaining why the private practice interest group is voicing serious concern about the continued profitability of psychological private practice (PASA, 1991). Clearly, the number of trained practitioners is insufficient for population needs, but skewed distribution of existing resources and services is also a major problem.

PSYCHOLOGY IN EDUCATIONAL SETTINGS

The privileged sector of the South African population has psychological services in education that are comparable to most First World countries (Donald, 1991). On the other hand, the vast educational, psychological and social needs of the nonprivileged majority are minimally provided for (Hickson & Kriegler, 1991a). The issue is not only the overall shortage of educational psychologists (a ratio of 1:12,000 of school-age population), but also the lack of social service personnel to serve this sector. The average ratio of these professionals for black education is 1:30,000, whereas for whites it is 1:2,750 (ratios for Asians and coloreds, as usual, fall somewhere in between). South Africa's school-age population currently stands at 8,647,000, of which 6,645,000 or 77 percent are black. Correcting the backlog and distorted distribution would require an immense expenditure—and that in a context in which basic educational needs (books, desks, amenities) are unmet (Nasson & Samuel, 1990). Furthermore, the existing model of service delivery has led to limited human and financial resources being exhausted on testing, with little, if any, benefit to testees (Kriegler, 1989). It is little wonder that school psychological services have been cut to the bone in Natal, with the other provinces likely to follow suit.

STRUCTURAL PROBLEMS IN MENTAL HEALTH SERVICES

According to Freeman (1992) and the Psychological Association of South Africa (PASA, 1989), the administration and provision of mental health is irrational, wasteful and fragmented. While overall there is a gross undersupply of services, there is overlap and even oversupply in certain areas. Intersectoral and interdepartmental cooperation is limited. Many of these problems are rooted in apartheid structures: fourteen departments of health, twenty-five racially divided regional welfare boards, and segregated hospitals and community services. Much the same may be said of school psychological and health services. There is a lack of coordination and integration between social, psychological and health services provided in hospital and clinic settings on the one hand, and school settings on the other. School psychological services are often dominated by nonregistered, pedagogically trained personnel who enjoy the protection of the educational departments.

Another problem is the medical hegemony in state services. Psychologists are virtually unrepresented at the level of decision making and planning (PASA, 1989; 1991). Any multidisciplinary team is automatically led by a psychiatrist. The first post for a psychologist in the Department of National Health's Chief Directorate for Mental Health is only now being advertised. It is hardly surprising that psychological services are neglected at the service level.

ATTITUDINAL BARRIERS TO EFFECTIVE MENTAL HEALTH SERVICES

The underrepresentation of culturally diverse clients in mental health services is not unusual (Sue & Sue, 1990). Some of the reasons for this problem are (1) most psychologists are white, middle-class and English- or Afrikaans-speaking, (2) generic characteristics of counseling and psychotherapy (individual-centered, verbal, separating physical and mental) and (3) factors related to communication style (such as proxemics, paralanguage and kinesics).

The effects of historical and current oppression, discrimination and racism also create psychological barriers to mental health services (Straker, 1986). Institutional racism in South Africa has fostered and sanctioned the enactment of discriminatory statutes, the selective enforcement of laws, and the blocking of economic opportunities and outcomes. Feelings of powerlessness, inferiority, subordination, deprivation, anger and rage are likely to persist. White people, including mental health workers, may be perceived as enemies until proven otherwise. Nor are (even the most well-meaning) psychologists immune from inheriting racist attitudes, beliefs, myths and stereotypes (Swartz, 1991).

PRESENT TRAINING PROGRAMS

Psychological training programs have often fostered cultural encapsulation. This term refers to (1) the substitution of model stereotypes for the real world, (2) the disregarding of cultural variations in dogmatic adherence to some universal notion of truth, and (3) the use of a technique-oriented definition of the counseling process (Sue & Sue, 1990). Few black, colored or Asian candidates apply for training in advanced programs. The Professional Board for Psychology recommends—but does not require—the inclusion of cross-cultural material or experience for accreditation of courses. Much of the problem resides in the lack of direction and the tedious process of developing new programs, especially as universities are already under considerable stress and staff are overloaded with research responsibilities (although much of the research does not escape the same criticism as pertains to training). The rationalization imperative may be the spark that fires the creativity to develop new options and directions.

FINANCING MENTAL HEALTH CARE

In conjunction with the likely proliferation of health maintenance organizations, preferred provider organizations, and individual practice associations (seeing that the managed care principle has been largely accepted by the health professions), future mental health care at the grassroots level may be funded through a National Health Insurance system. Inevitably, the services offered under managed care conditions will be limited to the so-called "bare bones," and some people will continue to buy services outside the system (De Gouveia, 1992; Freeman, 1992). In deciding how much to allocate to psychotherapy within managed care or state-funded structures, the cost benefits of psychotherapy should be borne in mind. The increased cost of adequately covering psychotherapy (especially on an outpatient basis) must be weighed against the reduction of medical costs associated with effective psychological treatment. Mentally unwell patients typically overutilize medical services. Many visits to primary care physicians are actually mental health related—some studies suggest the number may be 50 to 70 percent of a primary physician's caseload, depending upon how widely mental health is defined (De Gouveia, 1991).

Although it is much more difficult to determine the monetary value of preventive interventions than of curative strategies, recent studies estimate that approximately one-half of the deaths due to the ten most important causes of mortality in the United States may be associated with behaviorally related pathogens, such as alcohol abuse, overeating, risk-taking behavior, malnutrition and poor hygiene (PASA, 1991). In developing countries, there is a simultaneous increase in diseases related to prosperity and those associated with poverty and ignorance—malaria, tuberculosis, cholera and AIDS. It is estimated that some 100,000 to 300,000 people in South Africa are now AIDS carriers. If the population does not respond to health education, this pandemic will wipe out a large proportion of the population, not to mention the dire consequences it will have for the economy and the health services system (Steyn, undated). Counseling and educational psychological skills can especially help to achieve the change in emphasis to prevention and promotion that is advocated in the present government's future strategy for mental health in South Africa (Department of National Health and Population Development, 1991). However, development of psychological services and public recognition of their worth are prerequisites to psychologists taking their rightful place as indispensable members of the health-care team.

PSYCHOLOGY'S CATCH-22

The previous discussion takes us to the core of the profession's current dilemma: it is disempowered to position itself strategically in such a way as to ensure its relevance in a new South Africa. Organized psychology is paralyzed by divisions along ideological lines and between registration categories. Private practice is saturated in terms of demand and immersed in the individual model of service delivery. Moreover, a future government is unlikely to be more sympathetic to this group than the present one. In the schools, psychologists have lost posts—it will be no small task to convince the new educational planners that school psychology can mend its old, ineffectual ways. For example, the Directorate of National Health commented that the department does not employ psychologists because they are neither trained nor prepared to work "under a tree in Giyani." Yet students cannot be trained and motivated to twiddle their thumbs under that metaphorical tree: there are no job opportunities for psychologists in rural (or, for that matter, urban) community contexts. Indeed, a classic "catch-22" situation. One solution is for psychology to get its own house in order, but the state will also have to help. What is needed is concerted, affirmative action for psychology.

A CALL TO THE STATE

A Comprehensive and Coordinated National Strategy

It goes without saying that a coordinated and comprehensive national mental health policy and strategy will be needed if we are to attain the goal of "health for all by the year 2000" (Steyn, undated). Freeman (1992), arguing against the strong social work lobby for a separate Welfare Department, espouses a single Department of Health and Welfare. A strong and autonomous Division of Mental Health within such a department should contain subdivisions for medical, social, psychological and rehabilitative services, democratically structured so that the professions have equal power. However, some powerful mechanism will have to be devised to coordinate mental health policies and services in other contexts, where isolated psychologists have often been submerged in bureaucratic structures, especially in prisons, the police force and the armed forces. The possibility of two state departments jointly appointing personnel has been debated as a way of achieving coordination.

To address the accountability issue, government policy and planning should be advised by community and service groups convened for this purpose—a process already initiated by the existing department. However, lesser-organized groups should not be ignored—one should not be naive about the nature of popular democracy in a society that is torn by conflict and violence. Also, psychology should have strong representation in existing policy and decision-making bodies such as the Council for Health Policy, the Health Matters Committee and the Subcommittee on Mental Health (PASA, 1989; 1991), and in future bodies. This representation might help to ensure that psychology is mentioned alongside psychiatry when the training of health and mental health teams is planned. Present projections never mention a psychologist as a member of the mental health care team, although the stated objective is to move toward a community-based, preventive and health-promoting approach (Department of National Health and Population Development, 1991).

Posts and Training Opportunities in Health-Care Settings

More mental health posts in the state sector should be created—in psychiatric and general hospitals, and in community health centers. Many of these positions should be community, rather than hospital, based. To best utilize the high-level knowledge and skills of psychologists, they should function as consultants, planning and facilitating services performed by a variety of mental health workers in different institutional contexts, including traditional or indigenous healers. The creation of posts for district psychologists, similar to those in the British National Health Service, should be seriously considered (PASA, 1991). All practitioners choosing to remain outside full-time public health care should be encouraged to serve the underprivileged through part-time public service. Practitioners should also be encouraged to work in rural areas. The coercive measures suggested by Freeman (1992) will not be necessary if posts are provided and may only result in an exodus of professionals.

Training departments need settings and opportunities in which to practice appropriate and relevant knowledge and skills. The lack of posts for interns is one of the gravest problems facing psychology. Many of the existing posts have been phased out (e.g., at the HSRC's Center for Adult and Child Guidance and Pretoria University's Child Guidance Clinic, more than twenty internship positions have disappeared due to lack of financial support). Many interns are currently working without remuneration. To address the similar problem of unemployment and underutilization of psychologists in Mexico, an agreement was reached between the Department of Health and the National University. The university trains students, emphasizing community psychology, and in turn, students are guaranteed placement for practical training and an eventual permanent position in a health-care center. A similar project has been launched with great success in Cuba. The above examples are worth considering. Another possibility is to utilize psychologists on a national service basis to work in rural areas in hospitals and community health centers (PASA, 1991). Although PASA (1989) recommends that mental health care should be integrated into state primary health-care structures, neither health nor mental health services should be limited to hospital and clinic settings. Because more than one-half of the South African population is younger than sixteen years, and because the crisis in education poses arguably the most serious threat to future national well-being, the school is at least an equally important potential locus of delivery.

Psychology in the School of the Future

The *cri de coeur* for school improvement in South Africa will not be backed by more money (Nasson & Samuel, 1990; Nkomo, 1990). Yet major reform of the educational system can be the driving force to ameliorate social problems related to poverty, violence, illiteracy, AIDS, substance abuse, crime and family disintegration. Provided that (the presently elusive) cooperation between education and health departments can be established, educational structures can be integrated with health and human services (Kriegler, 1988). The embryo of this model is already in place in black schools in the form of teacher assistance teams known as Panels for Identification, Diagnosis and Assistance (PIDA) (Hickson & Kriegler, 1991a) and in the primary health care provided on a six-week basis at identified schools (Department of National Health and Population Development, undated). This projection of the school of the future has profound implications for community renewal, family preservation and the nature of delivery systems for health, human services and education.

Using the school as a locus of delivery for primary health, childcare, preschool and parent education, recreation and family counseling, as well as for traditional educational activities, will promote parent involvement, improved school climate, and community support of education. Identification of children and families in need of help is facilitated in a school setting, as is accessibility. Nor is "one-stop shopping" for primary and preventive health care and for mental health resources a bad idea for rural areas, where a number of schools in a particular area may be served from one central school (PASA, 1991).

A CALL TO THE PROFESSION

If psychology as a profession is to be valued by the state, it must demonstrate its good faith and ability to contribute to the betterment of the society's quality of life. This might be achieved by the following self-regenerating actions.

Confront the Political Nature of Counseling and Psychotherapy

For too long we have deceived ourselves into believing that the database that underpins the profession is morally, ethically, and politically neutral (Duckitt & Foster, 1991). The results have been (a) subtle perpetuation of the view that some groups are inherently pathological, (b) perpetuation of racially biased services, and (c) provision of an excuse to the profession for not taking social action to rectify inequities in the system (Foster, 1991; Sue & Sue, 1990; Swartz, 1991). This confrontation should be the first step in the self-healing process whereby the ideological schisms in organized psychology (not to mention the petty rivalries between "categories") may be transcended.

Jettison Inappropriate Assumptions in Training

The profession must move quickly to challenge positivistic conceptions of science and the white, Anglo-Saxon cultural assumptions permeating training programs (Tyler, 1989). It should never be assumed that the mere acquisition of cultural knowledge and the academic teaching of skills are enough to train an effective cross-cultural helper (Pedersen, 1988b). The curriculum must focus on immediate social problems and needs, each course containing a consciousness-raising component, an affective component, a knowledge component and a skills component. Several cross-cultural specialists have begun to develop white–identity development models that have implications for specific training goals (Sue & Sue, 1990).

Train Effective Cross-Cultural Psychologists

Psychology should develop licensing and credentialing procedures requiring culturally competent counselors qualified to work with all populations (Parker, 1988). There is a need to recognize indigenous psychology and cross-cultural counseling as important areas of specialization. Cross-cultural competence should, however, not only be seen as a separate field of psychology, but also as an integral part of competent counseling and psychotherapy. For this reason, cross-cultural psychology in South Africa should be somewhat like a development aid project; it will be truly successful only when it is no longer needed. It will succeed when it has been absorbed into mainstream psychology (Segall et al., 1990).

Deal with Racism, Sexism and Other Forms of Oppression

Psychologists must recognize that there is very little counseling or psychotherapy that is not cross-cultural, owing to the interplay between the social system variables determining the client's and the helper's cultural identities: gender; sexual orientation; age; socioeconomic status; educational level; lifestyle; work role; power position in society; natural support systems; functional roles such as handicaps; and formal and informal affiliations like church groups and political parties (Pedersen, 1988a). Psychologists must recognize that all forms of prejudice are mental health threats (Foster, 1991; Hickson & Kriegler, 1991a; Nell, 1990). The prescriptions and techniques to combat these hazards to well-being should be part of every psychologist's skills repertoire (Louw-Potgieter et al., 1991; Segall et al., 1990).

Train More, and More Effective, Psychologists

A much larger body of professional workers should be trained to offer basic mental health care in school, health and community contexts. Psychologists should be trained to be able to work in multidisciplinary teams in urban settings, but should also be able to work independently of the customary network of medical and paramedical professionals to whom anything "nonpsychological" is referred. The right to prescribe psychotropic medication will go a long way towards enhancing psychologists' status and independence, but should, of course, depend on the requisite training. Obviously, there is a strong need for psychology to attract more nonwhite persons to the profession, albeit a complex issue. Selection committees will have to find qualities and criteria for selecting students other than academic achievement, such as multilingualism and bicultural experience (Pedersen, 1988b).

Train Middle-Level Psychologists

Thousands of students attain a B.A. degree in psychology, yet cannot perform any useful mental health role—a costly and tragic waste. Problem solving and program design should be featured from the first year training level. Donald (1991) suggests the notion of a mental health worker whose skills are not simply a truncated version of the professional psychologist's, but specifically focused on community work. This relates to the concept of a community health worker as proposed by the Department of National Health and Population Development (undated), although the department seemed to have nurses in mind. Perhaps the answer is that communities must be allowed to recruit and determine the training needs of their own community health workers.

Devise Time and Cost-Effective Training Models

The cost effectiveness of integrated postgraduate training courses has been demonstrated at a number of universities. If these courses produce a psychologist who is a jack-of-all-trades but master of none, nothing has been gained. Combined training models necessitate that training commence at first-year level. The ideal of the gentleman-scholar, with a Bachelor of Arts degree upon which a smattering of professional skills may be grafted, has been abandoned by, most, if not all professions. The time has come for psychology to follow suit, although a directed undergraduate course will still include sociology, anthropology, philosophy, literature and other disciplines. The ideal should be to produce a graduate with an understanding of the bio-psycho-social dimensions of human behavior, with specialization coming later.

Create Alternative Training Contexts

The traditional university-cum-clinic context cannot provide sufficient opportunities to work with culturally different clients or to launch community based, multidisciplinary projects. A cross-cultural training institute or unit may be associated with a university or hospital, but it must be based in, and function in close consultation with, particular target communities. External sponsors will have to be found, as those most in need of proactive care cannot pay on a fee-for-service basis and few South African universities can afford nonsubsidized service-based training. The training must be wholly transcultural in the sense that a spectrum of scientific, professional and bureaucratic barriers must be transcended.

Students should be socialized to function and communicate effectively in multidisciplinary contexts.

Consult with Potential Clients, Consumers and Employers

It has been said that the most important function of the undergraduate courses in psychology has been to socialize thousands of potential clients into the culture of psychology. A process of consultation and negotiation will be needed to likewise sensitize the masses of South Africans who have never heard of psychology—a therapeutic culture must be created (Manganyi, 1991). Trainers will have to market the new professional roles envisaged for psychologists in the private and public sectors in which they want their graduates to be employed. This marketing should include informing and changing the attitudes of primary health-care teams, clergy and social workers. Marketing new professional roles and job creation for graduates should be seen as an integral part of the training responsibility.

Undertake Relevant, Responsible and Visible Research

Perhaps our fear of appearing unscientific has scared us away from the complex, the unknown, and even the significant (Sinha, 1989). Yet we cannot escape the moral and ethical responsibilities of research (Paranjpe, 1989). Research should focus not only on the effects of prejudice and oppression, but also on the sociocultural mechanisms operating to maintain them. The positive aspects of bi- and multiculturalism should be highlighted, along with the positive characteristics of culturally different groups. The image of psychology as being closely linked with clinical psychology or as a technique restricted to testing, may be altered by research focusing on social and cultural variables of individual behavior and directed toward solutions for major social problems (Segall et al., 1990). Research should be conducted in close cooperation with the communities who are to benefit from it. Longitudinal research projects should be undertaken in order to determine psychological trends and pathologies within the South African milieu.

Provide Acceptable and Accessible Services

Many clients may find it impossible to take time off from work to get to a hospital or clinic, and transportation difficulties may be insuperable. Twenty-four-hour community care services should be available and every community should have a crisis care center where the full spectrum of services is available. The case manager could be a paraprofessional, neighbor or unemployed person who receives an allowance for assisting people in getting to clinics, collecting their pensions, etc. The home visit is another outreach strategy historically used by social workers with very positive results. Indigenous languages should feature prominently in training courses. Services cannot be equitable and effective if they are not also acceptable and accessible (Health Matters Committee, 1992).

Utilize Natural Help-Giving Networks

Psychologists often operate under the ethnocentric assumption that counseling and psychotherapy never existed except in Western settings (Sinha, 1989; Sue & Sue, 1990). Consequently, traditional knowledge and natural help-giving networks have been delegitimized and stigmatized as superstition. Psychologists need to expand their perception of what constitutes mental health practices to include informal support systems (family, friends, community self-help programs and occupational networks). They should study, supplement and facilitate folk-healing methods and indigenous formal systems of therapy instead of attempting to destroy or replace them (Fuglesang, 1982; Hickson & Kriegler, 1991b).

Espouse Proactive Roles

In a consultant role, the psychologist would serve as resource person to mental health professionals and communities in developing programs. An outreach role requires that psychologists move out of their offices and into their clients' communities. For example, outreach and preventive programs could be delivered through the support of church and community organizations. An ombudsman role may involve identifying institutional policies and practices discriminating against an oppressed constituency (Sue & Sue, 1990). These new roles demand a shift from an individually oriented, curative model to a socially oriented, empowerment model: from the individual client to the family and its community network, from reactive to proactive interventions (Donald, 1991).

Adopt an Indirect Service Delivery Model

An "indirect service delivery model" means that psychologists work as consultants in relation to teachers, parents or others who have direct contact with the client. The basis of consultation is that it is a negotiated, mutual problem-solving relationship in which there are always two levels of psychological goal. One level is to reach solutions to the presenting problems, and the other is for the consultees to gain in psychological insights, skills and problem-solving ability so that they will have greater competence and confidence in dealing with future problems (Donald, 1991). In this context, paraprofessional and volunteer programs hold much promise, especially in rural areas (Heyman, 1983).

Adapt Family Therapy

Family therapy approaches are especially appropriate in working with various cultural groups. They highlight the importance of the family (versus the individual) as the unit of identity; they focus on resolution of concrete issues (versus abstractions); and place the therapist in an expert position (versus nondirective approaches). Family therapy attempts to understand the family's communication via reframing, versus self-disclosure of inner feelings, which is inappropriate in many black cultures. "Indigenization" means developing a psychology that is suited to the sociocultural soil (Paranjpe, 1989; Sinha, 1989). It would imply translation of goals and strategies into contemporary South African concepts of the family, which may include the living and the dead, the elders and the spirits (Fuglesang, 1982), and demands a bio-psycho-social approach (Tyler, 1989). A reconceptualization of what constitutes a healthy family (Mason & Rubenstein, 1989) will in turn enrich perceptions of white family dynamics.

Develop Systems Interventions

A paradigmatic shift in perceiving many psychosocial and educational problems as structural is required. A systems approach involves systemic analysis of a particular context (classroom, school, community) and the introduction of strategic input directed toward self-perpetuating change in the system as a whole. Provided this is done within a participatory framework, it has the potential to be extremely powerful in effecting far-reaching change (Donald, 1991) and is one of the ways to address the problem of anachronistic, elitist and cost-ineffective intervention modes endemic in psychology (De Gouveia, 1992).

CONCLUSION

Bulhan (1990) emphasizes that an Afrocentric psychology is not racially based—but rather a way of thinking and acting in the world. It is a psychology rooted in the history, legacy and ecology of Africa, which is holistic rather than analytic and interpersonal rather than intrapersonal (Fuglesang, 1982). This psychology "can be no other than an emancipatory one . . . which liberates people from internalized and institutionalized oppression" (Bulhan, 1990, p. 70). Finally, it is hoped that the new South Africa will be a healing culture, promoting the growth of all its citizens. In Mannheim's words "The continuous emergence of new human beings . . . teaches us both to forget that which is no longer useful and to covet that which has yet to be won" (cited in Jenks, 1982, p. 263).

Afterword: Hope and Reconciliation in the "New" South Africa

In South African history, the present represents an open moment. It suggests the promise of hope and reconciliation. The new South Africa can offer inclusion to all its people: the triumph of justice, the brotherhood of man and the dream realized.

The purpose of this book has been to use South Africa as a case example in order to better understand issues of multiculturalism. Many countries have had to contend with the difficulty of reconciling national unity with cultural diversity. In South Africa, variables such as the legacy of ethnic, linguistic or cultural groups must continue to be negotiated, as well as the existence of a regionalism associated with cultural identity. A major difficulty is that of socioeconomic conflict arising out of unemployment, race and class differences. Historically, policy approaches of the dominant white establishment to cultural pluralism have reflected a colonial mentality resulting in isolation and institutionalized racism. The creation of separate homelands for blacks and the official policy of apartheid reflect this stance. Because South Africa has officially sanctioned separate development for nondominant cultural groups, a well-developed sense of national unity that encompasses all peoples is sorely needed. Currently, South Africa is in the process of formulating a national ethos. Education will play a major role in creating this national culture.

Approaches to multicultural education in South Africa must avoid the extremes of the melting pot concept, which emphasized monoculturalism and the promotion of one set of exclusive values. The "salad bowl" approach, which emphasizes particularism and ethnic differences, must also be avoided due to its potential as a divisive element in an already bitterly divided and polarized society. Strict adherence to either one of these approaches could be counterproductive with respect to the building of national unity. Given South Africa's history and the destructive effects of apartheid, the educational curriculum must enrich and contribute to the creation of a national culture and national unity. Initially, a focus must be placed on global, rather than narrow and regional, interests. Because ethnic differences have been greatly overemphasized in South Africa, and because South Africa has not yet been successful in creating a national identity for all its people, the present strategy must be that of downplaying perceived differences. Efforts must be made to bind people together in a collective way. Once a national unity is achieved, a more critical perspective can be adopted that recognizes the difficulties of cultural diversity within an egalitarian social system. The larger goal of multicultural education in the beginning, however, should be to produce global thinkers and to promote tolerance. A world, rather than a parochial, perspective should be taught, and cultural learning interfused into a broader, universal context. In the South African context, it remains that education will be a major tool of reconciliation.

References

Abdi, Y. O. (1975). The prospect of psychology in Africa. *International Journal of Psychology, 100,* 224–234.

Ahia, C. E. (1984). Cross cultural counseling concerns. *Personnel and Guidance Journal, 62,* 339–341.

Alexander, N. (1990). Educational strategies for a new South Africa. In B. Nasson & J. Samuel (Eds.), *Education: From poverty to liberty* (pp. 166–180). Cape Town: David Philip.

Anonymous. (1986). Some thoughts on a more relevant or indigenous counseling psychology in South Africa: Discovering the socio-political context of the oppressed. *Psychology in Society, 5,* 81–89.

Appelgryn, A. (1991). Social comparison and relative deprivation: Perceived justice and intergroup attitudes. In D. Foster & J. Louw-Potgieter (Eds.), *Social psychology in South Africa* (pp. 237–272). Johannesburg: Lexicon.

Appiah, K. A. (1990). Racisms. In D. T. Goldberg (Ed.), *Anatomy of racism* (pp. 3–17). Minneapolis: University of Minnesota Press.

Balibar, E. (1990). Paradoxes of universality. In D. T. Goldberg (Ed.), *Anatomy of racism* (pp. 283–294). Minneapolis: University of Minnesota Press.

Barthes, R. (1990). Bichon and the blacks. In D. T. Goldberg (Ed.), *Anatomy of racism* (pp. 127–129). Minneapolis: University of Minnesota Press.

Bateson, G. (1944). Cultural determinants of personality. In J. Hunt (Ed.), *Personality and the behavior disorder* (pp. 723–730). New York: Roneoed Press.

Beckmann, J. L. (1991). Relevante onderwysersopleiding vir 'n multikulturele onderwysgemeenskap [Relevant teacher training for a multicultural education community]. *South African Journal of Education, 11* (4), 179–184.

Belkin, G. (1981). *Practical counseling in the schools.* Dubuque, Iowa: William C. Brown.

Bentley, A. M. & Miller, R. (1990). Resilient children and the cognitive consequences of poverty: A neo-Piagetian study with Zulu-speaking children. In Centre for Intergroup Studies, *The influence of violence on children: Occasional Paper No. 13* (pp. 185–195). Cape Town: Centre for Intergroup Studies.

Biesheuvel, S. (1987). Psychology: Science and politics: Theoretical developments and applications in a plural society. *South African Journal of Psychology, 17,* 1–8.

Binswanger, L. (1962). *Being-in the world: Selected papers.* New York: Basic Books.

Boating, R. (1983). African traditional education: A method of disseminating cultural values. *Journal of Black Studies, 13,* 321–336.

Botha, J. L., Du Plessis, P. J. J., Joubert, C. J., Botha, T. R., & Roos, S. G. (1975). *Jeugweer-baarheid* (Youth preparedness). Durban: Butterworths.

Bray, W. (1992). Human rights and education. *South African Journal of Education, 12*(1), 16–25.

Brislin, R. W. (1981). *Cross-cultural encounters.* New York: Pergamon.

Brislin, R. W. (1990). *Applied cross cultural psychology.* Newbury Park, Calif.: Sage.

Buhrmann, M. V. (1977). Xhosa diviners as psychotherapists. *Psychotherarpeia, 21,* 17–20.

Bulhan, H. A. (1990). Afrocentric psychology. Perspective and practice. In L. J. Nicholas & S. Cooper (Eds.), *Psychology and apartheid. Essays on the struggle for psychology and the mind in South Africa* (pp. 66–98). Johannesburg: Vision/Madiba.

Burlen, N. C. (1930). *Songs and tales from the dark continent.* New York: Schimmer.

Burman, S. (1986). The contexts of childhood in South Africa: An introduction. In S. Burman & P. Reynolds (Eds.). *Growing up in a divided society* (pp. 1–15). Evanston, Ill.: Northwestern University Press.

Burman, S. & Reynolds, P. (Eds.). (1986). *Growing up in a divided society.* Evanston, Ill.: Northwestern University Press.

Busia, K. A. (1963). The African world view. In J. Dracher (Ed.), *African Heritage* (pp. 100–125). New York: Crowell-Collier.

Carnoy, M. (1990). Socialist development and educational reform in Cuba 1959–1980. In B. Nasson & J. Samuel (Eds.), *Education: From poverty to liberty* (pp. 7–131). Cape Town: David Philip.

Center for Educational Research and Innovation (CERI). (1989). *One school, many cultures.* Paris: Organization for Economic Co-operation and Development (OECD).

Chombart de Lauwe, P. H. (1987). Technological domination and cultural dynamism. In Center for Educational Research and Innovation (CERI), *Multicultural education* (pp. 142–157). Paris: Organization for Economic Co-operation and Development (OECD).

Christie, P. (1990). Private open schools. In M. Nkomo (Ed.), *Pedagogy of domination: Toward a democratic education in South Africa* (pp. 179–198). Trenton, N.J.: Africa World Press.

Cilliers, S. P. (1971). *Education and status report on Colored peoples.* Johannesburg: Institute of Race Relations.

Cloete, N., Pillay, S. & Swart, A. (1986, September). *The pro-active counselor: Is neutrality possible?* Paper presented at the Annual Conference of the Society for Student Counseling in South Africa, Johannesburg.

Clowes, J. (1990). African self help: Our experiences of stress over the past 20 years. In Centre for Intergroup Studies, *The influence of violence on children: Occasional Paper No. 13* (pp. 62–66). Cape Town: Centre for Intergroup Studies.

Cock, J., Emdon, E. & Klugman, B. (1986). The care of the Apartheid child: An urban study. In S. Burman & P. Reynolds (Eds.), *Growing up in a divided society* (pp. 66–92). Evanston, Ill.: Northwestern University Press.

Coetzee, J. M. (1991). The mind of apartheid: Geoffrey Cronjé (1907–). *Social Dynamics, 17*(1), 1–15.

Cooper, S., Nicholas, L. J., Seedat, M. & Statman, J. M. (1990). Psychology and apartheid: The struggle for psychology in South Africa. In L. J. Nicholas & S. Cooper (Eds.), *Psychology and apartheid: Essays on the struggle for psychology and the mind in South Africa* (pp. 1–21). Johannesburg: Vision/Madiba.

Cross, M. & Chisholm, L. (1990). Roots of segregated schooling. In M. Nkomo (Ed.), *Pedagogy of domination: Toward a democratic education in South Africa* (pp. 43–74). Trenton, N.J.: Africa World Press.

Davie, E. (1990). Parental empowerment as a preventive strategy against violence. In Centre for Intergroup Studies, *The influence of violence on children: Occasional Paper No. 13* (pp. 206–209). Cape Town: Centre for Intergroup Studies.

Dawes, A. R. L. (1986). The notion of relevant psychology with particular reference to Africanist pragmatic initiatives. *Psychology in Society, 5,* 28–48.

Dawes, A. & Tredoux, C. (1990). The impact of political violence on the children of K.T.C. In Centre for Intergroup Studies, *The influence of violence on children: Occasional Paper No. 13* (pp. 67–86). Cape Town: Centre for Intergroup Studies.

Dawis, R. V. (1978). A paradigm and model for the cross-cultural study of counseling. *Personnel Guidance Journal, 51,* 463–467.

De Certeau, M. (1987). The management of ethnic resources: Schooling for diversity. In Center for Educational Research and Innovation (CERI), *Multicultural education* (pp. 164–188). Paris: Organization for Economic Co-operation and Development (OECD).

Degenaar, J. (1990). The concept of violence. In Centre for Intergroup Studies, *The influence of violence on children: Occasional Paper No. 13* (pp. 4–27). Cape Town: Centre for Intergroup Studies.

De Gouveia, A. D. (1991). *The medical cost-offset of psychotherapy.* Paper presented at the National Congress of the Psychological Association of South Africa, University of Pretoria, October 7–9, 1991.

De Gouveia, A. D. (1992). *The proposed amendments to the Medical Schemes Act and their implications for psychologist practitioners.* Pretoria: Psychological Association of South Africa.

De Klerk, W. A. (1975). *The puritans in Africa: A story of Afrikanerdom.* Harmondsworth: Penguin.

Delacampagne, C. (1990). Racism and the West: From praxis to logos. In D. T. Goldberg (Ed.), *Anatomy of racism* (pp. 83–88). Minneapolis: University of Minnesota Press.

Department of National Health and Population Development. (N.d.). *Strategy for community health workers.* Pretoria: Department of National Health and Population Development.

Department of National Health and Population Development. (1991). *The organisation of mental health services in the Republic of South Africa.* Pretoria: Department of National Health and Population Development.

Diaz-Guerrero, R. (1977). A Mexican psychology. *American Psychologist, 32,* 934–944.

Disasa, J. (1988). African Children's Attitude Toward Learning. *Journal of Multicultural Counseling and Development, 16,* 16–23.

Donald, D. (1991). Training needs in educational psychology for South African social and educational conditions. *South African Journal of Psychology, 21*(1), 38–44.

Donald, D. & Dawes, A. (1994). The way forward: Development research and intervention in contexts of adversity. In A. Dawes & D. Donald (Eds.), *Childhood in adversity* (pp. 261–271). Cape Town: David Philip.

Dowdall, T. (1990). Working with children and their families in civil conflict situations. In Centre for Intergroup Studies, *The influence of violence on children: Occasional Paper No. 13* (pp. 87–96). Cape Town: Centre for Intergroup Studies.

Duckitt, J. & Foster, D. (1991). Introduction to the special issue: race, social attitudes, and prejudice. *South African Journal of Psychology, 21*(4), 199–202.

Du Preez, J. M. (1983). *Africana, Afrikaner: Master symbols in South African school textbooks.* Alberton: Librarius.

Fanon, F. (1990). The fact of blackness. In D. T. Goldberg (Ed.), *Anatomy of racism* (pp. 108–126). Minneapolis: University of Minnesota Press.

Ferguson-Davie, C. J. (1952). *The early history of Indians in Natal.* Johannesburg: South African Institute of Race Relations.

Fitzgerald, M. (1980). *Urban community development in South Africa.* Johannesburg: McGraw-Hill.

Foster, D. (1986). The development of racial orientation in children: A review of South African research. In S. Burman & P. Reynolds (Eds.), *Growing up in a divided society* (pp. 158–183). Evanston, Ill.: Northwestern University Press.

Foster, D. (1991). "Race" and racism in South African psychology. *South African Journal of Psychology, 21*(4), 203–210.

Freeman, M. (1992). *Providing mental health care for all in South Africa: Structure and strategy.* Johannesburg: The Center for Health Policy, University of the Witwatersrand.

Fuglesang, A. (1982). *About understanding: Ideas and observations on cross-cultural communication.* Uppsala: Dag Hammarskjöld Foundation.

Gagiano, J. (1992). Probing the mind of white South Africa. *Democracy in Action, 6*(2), 10–11.

Gama, J. (1990). The impact of stress in our community: With a specific reference to children and youth. In Centre for Intergroup Studies, *The influence of violence on children: Occasional Paper No. 13* (pp. 53–61). Cape Town: Centre for Intergroup Studies.

Gardiner, M. (1990a). Alternative curricula. In M. Nkomo (Ed.), *Pedagogy of domination. Toward a democratic education in South Africa* (pp. 199–216). Trenton, N. J.: Africa World Press.

Gardiner, M. (1990b). People's English. In B. Nasson & J. Samuel (Eds.), *Education: From poverty to liberty* (pp. 159–165). Cape Town: David Philip.

Gbekobow, K. (1984). Counseling African children in the United States. *Elementary School Guidance and Counseling, 18,* 225–230.

Gibson, K. (1990). Case studies of children in political violence. In Centre for Intergroup Studies, *The influence of violence on children: Occasional Paper No. 13* (pp. 97–111). Cape Town: Centre for Intergroup Studies.

Gilroy, P. (1990). One nation under a groove. In D. T. Goldberg (Ed.), *Anatomy of racism* (pp. 263–282). Minneapolis: University of Minnesota Press.

Giordano, J. & Giordano, G. P. (1977). *The ethno-cultural factor in mental health: A lit-*

erature review and bibliography. New York: Institute on Pluralism and Group Identity.

Goldin, I. (1987). *Making race: The politics and economics of coloured identity in South Africa.* London: Longman.

Goldstone Commission. (1992). *The commission of inquiry regarding the prevention of public violence and intimidation.* Johannesburg: Government Printer.

Goodwin, J. (1985). *Cry Amandla! South African women and the question of power.* Johannesburg: Africana Publishing House.

Gordimer, N. (1954). Apartheid holiday. *Drum, 25,* 94–95.

Green, E. (1988). Can collaborative programs between biomedical and African indigenous health practitioners succeed? *Social Science and Medicine, 26,* 1126–1128.

Grenier, R. (1992). On the trail of America's paranoid class: Oliver Stone's JFK. *The National Interest,* Spring 1992, pp. 76–84.

Group for the Advancement of Psychiatry (1987). *Us and them: The psychology of ethnonationalism.* New York: Brunner/Mazel.

Gwalla-Ogisi, N. (1990). Special education in South Africa. In M. Nkomo (Ed.), *Pedagogy of domination: Toward a democratic education in South Africa* (pp. 217–288). Trenton, N.J.: Africa World Press.

Halstead, M. (1988). *Education, justice and cultural diversity: An examination of the Honeyford affair, 1984–85.* London: Falmer Press.

Harwood, A. (Ed.). (1981). *Ethnicity and medical care.* Cambridge, Mass.: Harvard University Press.

Health Matters Committee. (1992). *Agenda: Liaison forum for professional organizations.* Pretoria: Department of National Health and Population Development.

Hellman, E. (Ed.). (1949). *Handbook on race relations in South Africa.* London: Oxford University Press.

Hemmings, R. (1984). Mathematics. In A. Craft & G. Bardell (Eds.), *Curriculum opportunities in a multicultural society* (pp. 113–132). London: Harper & Row.

Herr, E. L. (1987). Cultural diversity from an international perspective. *Journal of Multicultural Counseling and Development, 15,* 99–110.

Hexham, I. (1981). *The irony of apartheid: The struggle for national independence of Afrikaner Calvinism against British Imperialism.* New York: Edwin Mellen.

Heyman, S. R. (1983). Problems in program development and the development of alternatives. In A. W. Childs & G. B. Melton (Eds.), *Rural psychology* (pp. 233–268). New York: Plenum Press.

Heyns, C. (1992). State-supported faith spells trouble. *Democracy in Action, 6*(1), 9–10.

Hicks, D. (1984). Geography. In A. Craft & G. Bardell (Eds.), *Curriculum opportunities in a multicultural society* (pp. 20–34). London: Harper & Row.

Hickson, J. & Kriegler, S. M. (1991a). Childshock: The effects of apartheid on the mental health of South Africa's children. *International Journal for the Advancement of Counseling, 14,* 141–154.

Hickson, J. & Kriegler, S. M. (1991b). The mission and role of psychology in a traumatized and changing society: The case of South Africa. *International Journal of Psychology, 26*(6), 783–793.

Hoare, C. H. (1991). Psychosocial identity development and cultural others. *Journal of Counseling and Development, 70,* 45–53.

Hodge, J. L. (1990). Equality: Beyond dualism and oppression. In D. T. Goldberg (Ed.), *Anatomy of racism* (pp. 89–107). Minneapolis: University of Minnesota Press.

Holdstock, T. L. (1979). Indigenous healing in S.A.: Neglected potential. *South African Journal of Psychology, 9,* 118–124.

Holdstock, T. L. (1981). Psychology in South Africa belongs to the colonial era: Arrogance or ignorance? *South African Journal of Psychology, 11,* 123–129.

Hughes, L. (1959). *Selected poems of Langston Hughes.* New York: Knopf.

Hutmacher, W. (1987). Cultural issues in educational policies: A retrospect. In Center for Educational Research and Innovation (CERI), *Multicultural education* (pp. 332–349). Paris: Organization for Economic Co-operation and Development (OECD).

Hyslop, J. (1990). Schools, unemployment and youth: Origins and significance of student and youth movements, 1976–1987. In B. Nasson & J. Samuel (Eds.), *Education: From poverty to liberty* (pp. 79–87). Cape Town: David Philip.

Inkatha Freedom Party. (1992, March 22). We say "thank you." *Sunday Star,* p. 7.

Institute of Race Relations. (1978). A survey of race relations in South Africa. Johannesburg: Institute of Race Relations.

Ivey, A. (1977). Toward a definition of the culturally effective counselor. *Personnel and Guidance Journal, 55,* 296–302.

Ivey, A. (1980). *Counseling and psychotherapy: Connections and application.* New York: Prentice Hall.

Ivey, A. (1986). Elements of a critical psychology. *Psychology in Society, 5,* 4–27.

James, W. (1992). Rattle dem bones. *Democracy in Action, 6*(2), 8–9.

Jansen, L. (1990). Education, pluralism and access to knowledge. In A. X. Cambridge & S. Feuchtwang (Eds.), *Antiracist strategies* (pp. 91–122). Aldershot: Avebury.

Jeffcoate, R. (1981). Curriculum planning in multicultural education. In A. James & R. Jeffcoate (Eds.), *The school in the multicultural society* (pp. 3–18). London: Harper & Row.

Jenks, C. (Ed.), (1982). *The sociology of childhood. Essential readings.* London: Batsford.

Jordaan, W. & Jordaan, J. (1984). *Man in context.* Johannesburg: McGraw-Hill.

Kagitcibasi, C. (1989). Why individualism/collectivism? In D. M. Keats, D. Munro & L. Mann (Eds.), *Heterogeneity in cross-cultural psychology* (pp. 66–74). Amsterdam: Swets & Zeitlinger.

Kakar, S. (1971). The theme of authority in social relations in India. *Journal of Social Psychology, 84,* 93–101.

Kakar, S. (1979). *Indian childhood: Cultural ideals and social reality.* Delhi, India: Oxford University Press.

Kashima, Y. (1989). Cultural conceptions of the person and individualism-collectivism: A semiotic framework. In D. M. Keats, D. Munro & L. Mann (Eds.), *Heterogeneity in cross-cultural psychology* (pp. 75–81). Amsterdam: Swets & Zeitlinger.

Kaufman, A. S., McLean, J. E., Ishikuma, T. & Moon, S. (1989). Integration of the literature on the intelligence of Japanese children and analysis of the data from a sequential-simultaneous perspective. *School Psychology International, 10*(3), 173–184.

Keto, C. T. (1990). Pre-industrial education policies and practices in South Africa. In M. Nkomo (Ed.), *Pedagogy of domination: Toward a democratic education in South Africa* (pp. 19–42). Trenton, N.J.: Africa World Press.

Khoapa, B. A. (1980). *The African personality.* Cleveland, Ohio: Case Western Reserve University Press.

Klaasen, E. (1990). The impact of violence on children. In Centre for Intergroup Studies,

The influence of violence on children: Occasional Paper No. 13 (pp. 49–52). Cape Town: Centre for Intergroup Studies.

Kleinman, A. C. (1980). *Patients and healers in the context of the borderland between anthropology, medicine and psychiatry.* Berkeley: University of California Press.

Kluckhohn, C. (1951). Values and value orientations in the theory of action. In T. Parsons & F. A. Shields (Eds.), *Toward a general theory of action* (pp. 388–433). Cambridge, Mass.: Harvard University Press.

Knowles, C. & Mercer, S. (1990). Feminism and antiracism: An exploration of the political possibilities. In A. X. Cambridge & S. Feuchtwang (Eds.), *Antiracist strategies* (pp. 61–90). Aldershot: Avebury.

Korman, M. (1974). National Conference on levels and patterns of professional training in psychology: Major themes. *American Psychology, 29,* 301–313.

Kriegler, S. M. (1988). Opleiding van opvoedkundige sielkundiges vir die bevordering van geestesgesondheid in Suid-Afrika. *Suid-Afrikaanse Tydskrif vir Sielkunde, 18*(3), 84–90.

Kriegler, S. M. (1989). The learning disabilities paradigm: Is it relevant in the South African context? *International Journal of Special Education, 4*(2), 165–171.

Kruger, T. M. D. (1974). Xhosa divining and contemporary psychotherapy—a reciprocal perspective. *Fort Hare Papers, 108,* 256–264.

Kuhn, L. (1990). The influence of violence on children: Epidemiological perspectives. In Centre for Intergroup Studies, *The influence of violence on children: Occasional Paper No. 13* (pp. 40–44). Cape Town: Centre for Intergroup Studies.

Kuper, H. (1958). The Indians of South Africa. In P. Smith (Ed.), *Africa in Transition* (pp. 115–127). London: Oxford University Press.

Lambley, P. (1980). *The psychology of apartheid.* Athens: University of Georgia Press.

Latakgomo, J. (1992, March 22). After the celebrations, the hangover. *Sunday Star,* p. 16.

Lazarus, S. (1986, October). *Training of psychologists for social responsibility in South Africa: A community psychology approach.* Paper presented at the Fourth National Congress of the Psychological Association of South Africa, Johannesburg.

Leach, G. (1989). *The Afrikaners.* Johannesburg: Southern.

Lelyveld, J. (1986). *Move your shadow. South Africa Black and White.* Johannesburg: Jonathan Ball.

Lemon, A. (1987). *Apartheid in transition.* Aldershot: Gower.

Le Roux, P. (1986). Growing up an Afrikaner. In S. Burman & P. Reynolds (Eds.), *Growing up in a divided society* (pp. 184–207). Evanston, Ill.: Northwestern University Press.

Livingstone, B. (1989). A study of apartheid education: Who shall do guidance? *Journal of Multicultural Counseling and Development, 17,* 171–179.

Louw, J. & Foster, D. (1991). Historical perspective: Psychology and group relations in South Africa. In D. Foster & J. Louw-Potgieter (Eds.), *Social psychology in South Africa* (pp. 55–90). Johannesburg: Lexicon.

Louw, L. & Kendall, F. (1986). *South Africa: The solution.* Bisho, Ciskei: Amagi Publications.

Louw-Potgieter, J. (1991). Language and identity. In D. Foster & J. Louw-Potgieter (Eds.), *Social psychology in South Africa* (pp. 315–341). Johannesburg: Lexicon.

Louw-Potgieter, J., Kamfer, L. & Boy, R. G. (1991). Stereotype reduction workshop. *South African Journal of Psychology, 21*(4), 219–224.

Malepa, M. (1990). The effects of violence on the development of young children in

Soweto. In Centre for Intergroup Studies, *The influence of violence on children: Occasional Paper No. 13* (pp. 45–48). Cape Town: Centre for Intergroup Studies.

Manganyi, N. C. (1991). *Treachery and innocence: Psychology and racial difference in South Africa.* Johannesburg: Ravan Press.

Maslow, A. H. (1971). *The farther reaches of human nature.* New York: Viking.

Mason, J. & Rubenstein, J. (1989). *Family therapy in South Africa today.* Congella: South African Institute of Marital and Family Therapy.

Matshekga, M. (1991). People's courts. *Lawyers for Human Rights* [special report], October 1991, pp. 39–42.

Mayer, P. & Mayer, I. (1990). A dangerous age: From boy to young man in Red Xhosa youth organisations. In P. Spencer (Ed.), *Anthropology and the riddle of the sphinx: Paradoxes of change in the life course* (pp. 35–44). London: Routledge.

Mbiti, J. S. (1970). *African religions and philosophy.* Garden City, N.Y.: Anchor Books.

McCormick, K. (1986). Children's use of language in District Six. In S. Burman & P. Reynolds (Eds.), *Growing up in a divided society: The contexts of childhood in South Africa* (pp. 288–307). Evanston, Ill.: Northwestern University Press.

McFadden, P. (1990). Freedom College. In M. Nkomo (Ed.), *Pedagogy of domination: Toward a democratic education in South Africa* (pp. 217–229). Trenton, N.J.: Africa World Press.

McGoldrick, M., Pearce, J. K. & Giordano, J. (1982). *Ethnicity and family therapy.* New York: The Guilford Press.

Meer, F. (1966). *Portrait of Indian South Africans.* Durban: Avon House.

Midgette, T. E. & Meggert, S. S. (1991). Multicultural counseling instruction: A challenge for faculties in the 21st century. *Journal of Counseling and Development, 70,* 136–141.

Moll, I. (1983). Answering the question: What is psychology? *Psychology in Society, 1,* 59–77.

Mukhopadhyay, A. (1984). Social sciences. In A. Craft & G. Bardell (Eds.), *Curriculum opportunities in a multicultural society* (pp. 35–54). London: Harper & Row.

Munro, D. (1989). Individualism and collectivism as consequences of the social process of self-categorization. In D. M. Keats, D. Munro & L. Mann (Eds.), *Heterogeneity in cross-cultural psychology* (pp. 82–91). Amsterdam: Swets & Zeitlinger.

Murphy, G. & Murphy, L. (1968). *Asian psychology.* New York: Basic Books.

Mynhardt, J. & Du Toit, A. (1991). Contact and change. In D. Foster & J. Louw-Potgieter (Eds.), *Social psychology in South Africa* (pp. 271–314). Johannesburg: Lexicon.

Naidoo, K. (1990). Student resistance. In M. Nkomo (Ed.), *Pedagogy of domination. Toward a democratic education in South Africa* (pp. 121–146). Trenton, N.J.: Africa World Press.

Nasson, B. (1990). Redefining inequality: Education reform and the state in contemporary South Africa. In B. Nasson & J. Samuel (Eds.), *Education: From poverty to liberty* (pp. 1–6). Cape Town: David Philip.

Nasson, B. & Samuel, J. (1990). Introduction. In B. Nasson & J. Samuel (Eds.), *Education: From poverty to liberty* (pp. 1–6). Cape Town: David Philip.

Nduka, O. (1980). Moral education in the changing traditional societies of Sub-Saharan Africa. *International Review of Education, 26,* 153–170.

Nell, V. (1990). Oppression, interpersonal violence, and the psychology of colonialism. In L. J. Nicholas & S. Cooper (Eds.), *Psychology and apartheid. Essays on the struggle for psychology and the mind in South Africa* (pp. 125–139). Johannesburg: Vision/ Madiba.

Nixon, J. (1985). *A teacher's guide to multicultural education.* London: Basil Blackwell.

Nkomo, M. (1990). Post-apartheid education. In M. Nkomo (Ed.), Pedagogy of domination. *Toward a democratic education in South Africa* (pp. 291–323). Trenton, N.J.: Africa World Press.

Outlaw, L. (1990). Toward a critical theory of "race." In D. T. Goldberg (Ed.), *Anatomy of racism* (pp. 58–82). Minneapolis: University of Minnesota Press.

Padilla, A. M., Ruiz, R. A. & Alveraz, R. (1975). Community mental health services for the Spanish-speaking-surnamed population. *American Psychologist, 30,* 892–905.

Paranjpe, A. C. (1989). Towards a pluralist approach to psychology: A metatheoretical critique of the unity of science model. In D. M. Keats, D. Munro & L. Mann (Eds.), *Heterogeneity in cross-cultural psychology* (pp. 41–53). Amsterdam: Swets & Zeitlinger.

Parker, W. M. (1988). *Consciousness-raising. A primer for multicultural counseling.* Springfield, Ill.: Charles C. Thomas.

Parker, W., Valley, M. & Geary, C. (1986). Acquiring cultural knowledge for counselors in training: A multifaceted approach. *Counselor Education and Supervision, 26,* p. 65.

PASA (1989). *Mental health in South Africa.* Report by the Council Committee: Mental Health. Pretoria: Psychological Association of South Africa.

PASA (1991). *Memorandum ten opsigte van samespreking tussen SVSA en Minister Rina Venter* (Memorandum regarding talks between PASA and Minister Rina Venter). Pretoria: Psychological Association of South Africa.

Paulston, C. B. (1987). Linguistic consequences of ethnicity and nationalism in multilingual settings. In Center for Educational Research and Innovation (CERI), *Multicultural education* (pp. 264–297). Paris: Organization for Economic Co-operation and Development (OECD).

Pauw, J. (1991). *In the heart of the whore: The story of apartheid's death squads.* Halfway House: Southern Africa Press.

Pedersen, P. B. (1978a). Asian personality theory. In R. J. Corsini (Ed.), *Innovative Psychotherapies* (pp. 367–397). New York: Wiley.

Pedersen, P. B. (1978b). Four dimensions of cross-cultural skill in counselor training. *Personnel and Guidance Journal, 56,* 480–484.

Pedersen, P. B. (1985). Cross-cultural counseling: U.S. perspectives. In R. Samuda (Ed.), *Cross-Cultural Counseling: International Perspectives* (pp. 71–83). Toronto: C. J. Hogrefe.

Pedersen, P. B. (1987). Ten frequent assumptions of cultural bias in counseling. *Journal of Multicultural Counseling and Development, 1,* 16–24.

Pedersen, P. B. (1988a). *A handbook for developing multicultural awareness.* Alexandria, Virginia: American Association for Counseling and Development.

Pedersen, P. B. (1988b). Intercultural training of mental health providers. In D. Landis & R. Brislin (Eds.), *Handbook of Intercultural Training* (pp. 325–350). New York: Pergamon Press.

Pedersen, P. B. (1991). Multiculturalism as a generic approach to counseling. *Journal of Counseling and Development, 70,* 6–12.

Pieterse, H. (1992). Afrikaans: Gister en vandag (Afrikaans: Yesterday and tomorrow). *Unisa-Bulletin, 17* (2), 6–7.

Pillay, A. L. (1987). Models of consultation in the practice of paediatric psychology. *Psychotherapeia, 14* (3), 19–23.
Pillay, P. N. (1990). The development and underdevelopment of education in South Africa. In B. Nasson & J. Samuel (Eds.), *Education: From poverty to liberty* (pp. 30–47). Cape Town: David Philip.
Platzky, L. & Walker, C. (1985). *The surplus people: Forced removals in South Africa.* Johannesburg: Ravan.
Ponterretto, J. G. & Casas, J. M. (1991). *Handbook of racial/ethnic minority counseling research.* Springfield, Ill.: Charles C. Thomas.
Prabhu, P. N. (1954). *Hindu social organization.* Bombay: Satsangi.
Psychology in Society Editorial (1983). *Psychology in Society, 5,* 1–20.
Psychology in Society Editorial (1986). *Psychology in Society, 1,* 1–20.
Ramphele, M. (1994). Foreword. In A. Dawes & D. Donald (Eds.), *Childhood and adversity* (pp. v–vi). Cape Town: David Philip.
Rapport, M. (1992, March 22). Letter from F.W. de Klerk to fellow South Africans. *Sunday Star,* p. 5.
Reilly, P. & Hofmeyr, F. (1983). *Pre-primary education in the Republic of South Africa.* Pretoria: Human Science Research Council.
Retief, A. I. (1986). *Theories of culture and environment: Common themes.* Paper presented at the Fourth National Congress of the Psychological Association of South Africa, Johannesburg.
Robertson, B. (1990). The influence of violence on children. In Centre for Intergroup Studies, *The influence of violence on children: Occasional Paper No. 13* (pp. 135–140). Cape Town: Centre for Intergroup Studies.
Roskam, K. (1992). Racist parties—what fate? *Democracy in Action, 6* (1), 6–7.
Saayman, G. (1990). Introduction. In G. Saayman (Ed.), *Modern South Africa in search of a soul. Jungian perspectives on the wilderness within* (pp. 1–17). Boston: Sigo Press.
Sadlak, M. J. & Ibrahim, F. A. (1986). *Cross-cultural counselor training: Impact on counselor effectiveness and sensitivity.* Paper presented at the 94th Annual Meeting of the American Psychological Association, Washington, D.C. (Division 17).
Samoff, J. (1990). Educational reform in Tanzania: Schools, skills and social transformation. In B. Nasson & J. Samuel (Eds.), *Education: From poverty to liberty* (pp. 132–140). Cape Town: David Philip.
Samuel, J. (1990). The state of education in South Africa. In B. Nasson & J. Samuel (Eds.), *Education: From poverty to liberty* (pp. 17–29). Cape Town: David Philip.
Sarason, S. B. (1984). If it can be studied or developed, should it be? *American psychologist, 39,* 477–485.
Schmidt, D. (1992). An obsession with tolerance? *Democracy in Action, 6*(2), 12–13.
Schuring, G. (1992). *A language policy for South Africa.* Paper delivered at the International Conference on Language and Law, Pretoria, April 27–30, 1992.
Schwartz, A. J. (1985). The schools and socialization. New York: Harper & Row.
Seelye, H. N. (1988). *Teaching culture. Strategies for intercultural communication.* Lincolnwood, Ill.: National Textbook Company.
Segall, M. H., Dason, P. B., Berry, J. W. & Poortinga, Y. A. (1990). *Human behavior in global perspective: An introduction to cross-cultural psychology.* New York: Pergamon.
Simpson, G. (1992, March 22). The real results behind the referendum roundabout. *Sunday Star,* p. 16.
Sinha, D. (1989). Cross-cultural psychology and the process of indigenization: A second

view from the third world. In D. M. Keats, D. Munro & L. Mann (Eds.), *Heterogeneity in cross-cultural psychology*. Amsterdam: Swets & Zeitlinger.

Smith, D. (1980). The impact of world views on professional life-styling. *Personnel and Guidance Journal, 58,* 584–587.

Smith, E. (1974). *Evolution and continuing presence of the African oral tradition in black America.* Ph.D. dissertation, University of California, Irvine.

Spencer, P. (1990). The riddled course: Theories of age and its transformations. In P. Spencer (Ed.), *Anthropology and the riddle of the sphinx: Paradoxes of change in the life course* (pp. 1–26). London: Routledge.

Spoonley, P. (1988). *Racism and ethnicity.* Auckland: Oxford University Press.

Steyn, D. P. (1985). *Relevant psychology in practice.* Paper presented at the Third National Congress of the Psychological Association of South Africa, Johannesburg.

Steyn, H. J. (N.d.). Executive summary by Dr. H. J. Steyn, Deputy Director-General of the Department of National Health and Population Development-RSA. Pretoria: Department of National Health and Population Development.

Steyn, J. C. & Viljoen, C. M. (1991). Enkele perspektiewe op die problematiek van skoolkurrikulumvernuwing vir multikulturele Suid-Afrika (Multiple perspectives on the problem of school curriculum transformation for a multicultural South Africa). *South African Journal of Education, 11*(4), 244–247.

Straker, G. (1986). *Black township refugees: Problems in treatment.* Unpublished manuscript (pp. 1–19). Department of Psychology, University of the Witwatersrand, Johannesburg.

Straker, G., Moosa, F. & Sanctuaries Counselling Team (1990). Post-traumatic stress disorder: A reaction to state-supported child abuse and neglect. In Centre for Intergroup Studies, *The influence of violence on children: Occasional Paper No. 13* (pp. 112–134). Cape Town: Centre for Intergroup Studies.

Strumpfer, D. J. W. (1981). Towards a more socially responsive psychology. *South African Journal of Psychology, 11,* 19–28.

Sue, D. W. (1978). Counseling across cultures. *Personnel and Guidance Journal, 56,* 450–452.

Sue, D. W. & Sue, D. (1977). Barriers to effective cross-culture counseling. *Journal of Counseling Psychology, 24,* 420–429.

Sue, D. W. & Sue, D. (1990). *Counseling the culturally different.* Theory and practice (2nd ed.). New York: John Wiley.

Sullivan, H. S. (1953). *Conceptions of modern psychiatry.* New York: Norton.

Surya, N. (1969). Ego structure in the Hindu joint family. Some considerations. In W. Caudell and T. Y. Lin (Eds.), *Mental Health Research in Asia and the Pacific.* Honolulu: East-West Center Press.

Swartz, L. (1991). The reproduction of racism in South African health care. *South African Journal of Psychology, 21*(4), 240–246.

Swartz, S., Dowdall, T. & Swartz, L. (1986). Clinical psychology and the 1985 crisis in Cape Town. *Psychology in Society, 5,* 131–138.

Taylor, C. A. (1991). Koöperatiewe leer—'n vorm van kompenseringsonderwys in 'n tegnologiese era (Co-operative learning—a form of compensatory education in a technological era). *South African Journal of Education, 11*(4), 144–147.

Theron, E. & Du Toit, J. B. (1977). *Kortbegrip van die Theron-verslag* (Short understanding of the Theron Report). Cape Town: Tafelberg.

Thompson, R. T. (1974). *African and in motion.* Los Angeles: University of California Press.

Tidwell, R. (1980). Counseling in a multicultural school setting. *Journal of Non-White Concerns, 9,* 84–90.

Triandis, H. C. (1980). Introduction to handbook of cross-cultural psychology. In H. C. Triandis & W. Lambert (Eds.), *Handbook of cross-cultural psychology,* Vol. 1 (pp. 1–21). Boston: Allyn & Bacon.

Tucker, C. M., Chennault, S. A. & Mulkerne, D. J. (1981). Barriers to effective counseling with blacks and therapeutic strategies for overcoming them. *Journal of Non-White Concerns, 9,* 69–76.

Turton, R. W. (1986). Bourgeois counseling and working class clients: Some problems and political implications. *Psychology in Society, 6,* 85–100.

Tyler, F. B. (1989). A psychological perspective on cross-cultural unity in psychology. In D. M. Keats, D. Munro & L. Mann (Eds.), *Heterogeneity in cross-cultural psychology* (pp. 54–65). Amsterdam: Swets & Zeitlinger.

Van der Post, Sir Lourens (1990). Foreword. In G. Saayman (Ed.), *Modern South Africa in search of a soul. Jungian perspectives on the wilderness within.* Boston: Sigo Press.

Van Schoor, W. A. (1986). *Intergroup counseling: Problems and possible solutions.* Paper presented at the Annual Conference of the Society for Student Counseling in Southern Africa. Johannesburg.

Van Zyl, A. (1990). The prevalence of psychiatric disorders in children and adolescents. In Centre for Intergroup Studies, *The influence of violence on children: Occasional Paper No. 13* (pp. 149–184). Cape Town: Centre for Intergroup Studies.

Vontress, C. E. (1969). Culture barriers in the counseling relationship. *Personnel and Guidance Journal, 48,* 11–17.

Vontress, C. E. (1979). Cross-cultural counseling: An existential approach. *Personnel and Guidance Journal, 58,* 117–121.

Vontress, C. E. (1983). An existential approach to cross-cultural counseling. *Counseling and Values, 28,* 2–12.

Washington, V. & Lee, C. C. (1981). Teaching and counseling the Black child: A systematic analysis for the 1980's. *Journal of Non-White Concerns, 10,* 60–66.

Wilkins, I. & Strydom, H. (1978). *The super-Afrikaners.* Johannesburg: Jonathan Ball.

Wilson, F. & Ramphele, M. (1989). *Uprooting poverty. The South African Challenge.* Cape Town & Johannesburg: David Philip.

Wood, A. (1984). Religious Education. In A. Craft & G. Bardell (Eds.), *Curriculum opportunities in a multicultural society* (pp. 55–70). London: Harper & Row.

Worrall, M. (1981). Multiracial Britain and the Third World: Tensions and approaches in the classroom. In A. James & R. Jeffcoate (Eds.), *The school in the multicultural society* (pp. 178–187). London: Harper & Row.

Wrenn, C. G. (1962). The culturally-encapsulated counselor. *Harvard Educational Review, 32,* 444–449.

Wrenn, C. G. (1985). Afterword: The culturally encapsulated counselor revisited. In P. B. Pedersen (Ed.), *Handbook of cross-cultural counseling therapy* (pp. 323–329). Westport, Conn.: Greenwood Press.

Zahran, D. (1979). *The religion, spirituality and thought of traditional Africa.* Chicago: University of Chicago Press.

Zec, P. (1981). Multicultural education: What kind of relativism is possible? In A. James & R. Jeffcoate (Eds.), *The school in the multicultural society* (pp. 29–44). London: Harper & Row.

Name Index

Subject Index

About the Authors

JOYCE HICKSON received her Ph.D. in counseling from Mississippi State University. Dr. Hickson spent six years in the southern Africa region where she was a Professor with the University of the Witwatersrand in Johannesburg and worked as a consultant to several African nations. She currently serves as Chair of the Department of Counseling and Clinical Programs at Columbus College in Columbus, Georgia.

SUSAN KRIEGLER is Associate Professor of Education Psychology and Special Education at the University of Pretoria, South Africa. She is a recipient of the Psychological Association of South Africa's Presidents Award for her contribution to renewal in the profession.

ISBN 0-313-28554-3

90000>

EAN

9 780313 285547

HARDCOVER BAR CODE